Nursing in Child and Adolescent Mental Health

Nisha Dogra and Sharon Leighton

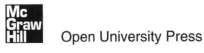
Open University Press

Open University Press
McGraw-Hill Education
McGraw-Hill House
Shoppenhangers Road
Maidenhead
Berkshire
England
SL6 2QL

email: enquiries@openup.co.uk
world wide web: www.openup.co.uk

and Two Penn Plaza, New York, NY 10121-2289, USA

First published 2009

A catalogue record of this book is available from the British Library

ISBN-13: 978-0-33-523463-9 (pb) 978-0-33-523462-2 (hb)
ISBN-10: 0335234631 (pb) 0335234623 (hb)

Library of Congress Cataloging-in-Publication Data
CIP data applied for

Typeset by RefineCatch Limited, Bungay, Suffolk
Printed in the UK by Bell and Bain Ltd, Glasgow

Fictitious names of companies, products, people, characters and/or data that may be used herein (in case studies or in examples) are not intended to represent any real individual, company, product or event.

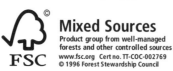

Mixed Sources
Product group from well-managed forests and other controlled sources
www.fsc.org   Cert no. TT-COC-002769
© 1996 Forest Stewardship Council

The **McGraw·Hill** Companies

Nursing in Mental Health

Praise for this book

"Nurses have a key role to play within the Child and Adolescent Mental Health Team. Yet there are few textbooks devoted to the specialist and advanced roles which many undertake within this field of practice. This text will fill the void addressing legal and ethical issues while focusing upon clinical practice and the application of theoretical concepts."
Fiona Smith, Adviser in Children's and Young People's Nursing, Royal College of Nursing

"It includes contributions from a range of experts who bring their insights from work across many settings. The case vignettes inserted represent a broad range of childhood problems, but this book is not prescriptive about nursing care. On the contrary, readers are encouraged to consider for every child the wider contexts of child development, parenting, multi-agency collaboration, safeguarding and the evaluation of outcomes."
Woody Caan, Department of Child & Family Health, Anglia Ruskin University, Cambridge, UK

"This book considers the range of skills and roles that nurses now undertake within specialist CAMHS, it provides a good basic introduction for nurses and clinicians from other disciplines. Discussion around medication management as part of a nurse's extended role is timely and will be of particular use to those considering this option within their practice. The text is easily accessible, utilising case studies to enhance learning. The inclusion of research and audit helps raise the need not only for nurses to be more involved in research but also the need for clinicians to evaluate their practice. I would recommend this text to clinicians new to CAMHS."
Sharon Pagett, Senior Lecturer, Mental Health (CAMHS), University of Central Lancashire, UK

Contents

The editors

Dr Nisha Dogra is a senior lecturer and honorary consultant in child and adolescent psychiatry at the University of Leicester. She has published in child mental health, diversity and medical education. She is an experienced child psychiatrist and has been involved in multi-disciplinary working and training. Nisha is the course director of the Postgraduate Certificate/Diploma/MSc in Child and Adolescent Mental Health at the University of Leicester, a course she established and which is becoming increasingly popular with nurses.

Dr Sharon Leighton is a nurse consultant in child and adolescent mental health at South Staffordshire and Shropshire Healthcare NHS Trust. She has worked in CAMHS since 1989. She holds honorary posts at the School of Health, Staffordshire University and The Greenwood Institute of Child Health, Leicester University, and is involved in research and teaching activities at both universities. Sharon was a member of the Guideline Development Group for the NICE Guidelines on Depression in Children and Young People (2003–5). She is a member of the Advisory Board for the *Journal of Child & Adolescent Mental Health*.

The contributors

Dr Laurence Baldwin, nurse consultant, children and young people, Derbyshire Mental Health Services NHS Trust and special lecturer, University of Nottingham.

Dr P. Mani Das Gupta, senior lecturer and learning & teaching fellow, Faculty of Sciences, Department of Psychology, Staffordshire University.

Dee Davies, now retired, but was formerly (until August 2008) Head of Nursing, Leicestershire Partnership NHS TRust.

Viki Elliot, specialist adoption nurse, child and adolescent mental health services, Leicestershire Partnership NHS Trust.

Clay Frake, clinical nurse specialist, child and adolescent mental health services, Leicestershire Partnership NHS Trust.

Neil Hemstock, charge nurse, Oakham House child and adolescent mental health services, Leicestershire Partnership NHS Trust.

Dr Michael Hodgkinson, consultant psychologist, child and adolescent mental health services, Leicestershire Partnership NHS Trust.

Sarah Hogan, nurse consultant, child and adolescent mental health services, Northampton, regional child and adolescent mental health services development manager.

Cath Kitchen, Hospital and Outreach Education, Northamptonshire.

Professor Peter Nolan, professor of mental health nursing, University of Staffordshire.

Teresa Norris, senior charge nurse, learning disability team, child and adolescent mental health services, Leicestershire Partnership NHS Trust.

Ged Rogers, head of corporate training, St Andrew's Healthcare, Northampton.

Noreen Ryan, nurse consultant, child and adolescent mental health services, Royal Bolton Hospital NHS Foundation Trust.

Mervyn Townley, consultant nurse, Gwent Specialist Child and Adolescent Mental Health Service, Aneurin Bevan Local Health Board, Wales. Fellow, Welsh Institute for Health and Social Care, Faculty of Health, Sport and Science, University of Glamorgan.

Professor Panos Vostanis, professor and honorary consultant, child and adolescent psychiatrist, University of Leicester.

Professor Richard Williams, professor of mental health strategy, Welsh Institute for Health and Social Care, Faculty of Health, Sport and Science, University of Glamorgan. Honorary professor of child and adolescent mental health, Lancashire School of Postgraduate Medicine, University of Central Lancashire and consultant child and adolescent psychiatrist, Aneurin Bevan Local Health Board, Wales.

Acknowledgements

Both Nisha and Sharon would like to thank all the contributors to this book; it goes without saying we could not have done it without you.

Special thanks to Jo Welch for the administrative support provided in putting the final version together. Thanks also to Clay Frake, Neil Hemstock, Khalid Karim, Dr Christian Dunn and Smita Patel for reading various drafts. The feedback provided was most helpful.

Introduction

Nisha Dogra and Sharon Leighton

This book has proved an interesting and challenging project. While both of us are very aware of the important role that nurses play in delivering specialist and generic care to children and young people with mental health problems, the written evidence to support their contribution is limited. Writing this book has helped us appreciate even more the importance of recognizing and valuing the specialist role of all mental health professionals in child and adolescent mental health services (CAMHS). Although the primary audience is nurses, others in the multi-disciplinary team may also find the book useful.

The aim of this book

In considering what would form the key text, we took a decision that the focus of this book would not be information regarding specific mental disorders or problems that children may experience. There are already many excellent books available, written at different levels. We wanted to write a book that used the academic evidence available but was also grounded in the reality of clinical practice. We thought it was important to produce a text that looked at the various roles CAMH nurses fulfil and that also considered how we might enable those roles to be undertaken with confidence.

The scale of the problem

It is estimated that between 10 and 20 per cent of children and young people experience mental health problems (Meltzer *et al.* 2000). The rates are even higher for children and young people in vulnerable groups such as looked-after children, homeless children and refugees. Only a minority of these children receive the services they need. Nurses play an integral role in CAMHS, helping to deliver services that reduce suffering for children and young people and enabling them to achieve their potential. The numbers of nursing staff in CAMHS are rising, with an increasing diversity of roles. We were keen to write a textbook especially for nurses that would help them to fulfil their roles and offer them differing perspectives to reflect upon. We consider the specific role of nurses in several key areas of their clinical practice and professional working life. The reader is provided with opportunities to engage with the text through interactive exercises and where relevant each chapter includes boxes to highlight key points, along with case scenarios and clinical examples to illustrate how the theoretical aspects apply in practice. We suggest that you undertake the exercises and case scenarios with colleagues. Wherever possible we have related the exercises and scenarios to the literature available, however, unfortunately, in many areas specific literature relating to both CAMH nurses and child mental health per se is often lacking and in such cases (e.g. stigma, audit, clinical governance) we have referred to the relevant associated literature.

CAMH nursing as an art and a science

In this introduction we want to assert that we believe that mental health nursing is both an art and a science. We will introduce specialist child and adolescent mental health services (SCAMHS) and CAMH nursing. While the work of school nurses, health visitors, children's nurses and learning disability nurses involves CAMHS provision, and the principles discussed here are applicable in all areas, the main focus of this discussion is on specialist CAMH nurses working at Tiers 2–3 (HAS 1995).

The process of nursing

Traditional definitions classify nursing as a practical process involving assessment, planning, intervention, recording, evaluation and decision-making. Roper *et al.* (1986) equate nursing with problem-solving. However, this approach is problematic as it essentially constrains the many varied contexts in which nursing occurs (Varcoe 1996). Crow *et al.* (1995) take another stance by identifying differences in areas of specialism. Here, domain-specific knowledge is applied by nurses within the context of their work and in terms of levels of novice and expert practice. However, defining nursing solely as a procedure-driven process can be seen to under-mine the role by dehumanizing it (Rosenbrock 1987). Paterson and Zderad state that 'the mean-ing of nursing as a living human act is in the act itself . . . nursing is a response to the human situation . . . one human being needs a kind of help and another gives it' (1988: 11).

Focusing specifically on mental health nursing in the UK, Norman and Ryrie (2005) identify two current polarized positions: interpersonal relations (the artists) and evidence-based practice (the scientists). In practice, mental health nurses are influenced by both, although they may favour one approach over the other. The interpersonal relations approach has its roots in Peplau's (1952) identification of mental health nursing as an interpersonal, therapeutic process. Current development is seen in the emerging concept of recovery and the development of the *tidal model* (Buchanan-Barker and Barker 2008). Meanwhile, the development of evidence-based health care has produced a group of '*expert*' nurse practitioners keen to take on many tasks previously associated with psychiatry (e.g. prescribing medication, detaining under the Mental Health Act – see Norman and Ryrie 2005). A clinical example demonstrating that a middle road is helpful can be seen in the provision of grief therapy for adolescents experiencing complicated grief (Leighton 2008).

Nursing within CAMHS

The role and history of nursing in CAMHS

Defining the role of mental health nurses in CAMHS is more difficult than one might antici-pate. CAMHS is considered to be a young health care specialism with its roots in the child guidance movement (Williams and Gale 2003). Until the mid-1990s service provision depended more on local professional inspiration and commitment than on explicit policy (Williams and Gale 2003). However, it is now broadly recognized that many mental health problems have their origins in childhood (Heginbotham and Williams 2005). Therefore, since the 1990s, CAMHS within the UK have been given increasing attention – for example, through the work of the NHS Health Advisory Service, and the consideration of the Welsh Assembly and the Departments of Health and Education (Heginbotham and Williams 2005).

Nursing was not a key discipline in CAMHS until the advent of adolescent psychiatric inpatient units in the late 1960s and early 1970s. Initially, the majority of nurses worked in inpatient services (Williams and Gale 2003). Although the number of inpatient CAMHS has declined in the last two decades, the number of nurses working in community-based CAMHS has grown enormously. In 2006 there were 9,705 clinical staff employed in specialist CAMHS, with nurses representing the largest percentage of the workforce (28 per cent) (DoH and DfCSF 2007).

The roles nurses play

Nurses in CAMHS provide a range of psychotherapeutic interventions to children and adolescents, and their families or carers. These include cognitive behavioural therapy (CBT), dialectical behaviour therapy (DBT) and family therapy. Furthermore, CAMH nurses are involved in multi-agency projects, working with children, young people and their families in various capacities, such as primary mental health workers, community psychiatric nurses, counsellors and advisers in school and social settings, and also in the capacity of research and project coordinators. Nurses provide specialist interventions with depressed, psychotic or anxious young people, adolescents with eating disorders and children who have been abused or traumatized. Some nurses specialize in interventions such as parenting programmes, consultation and the management of deliberate self-harm. With proved effectiveness, clinical activity translates into nursing practice guidance and interventions.

Nevertheless, CAMH nurses struggle to define their position. CAMH nursing is seen as holistic, eclectic and not fully appreciated by other disciplines (Limerick and Baldwin 2000; Leighton et al. 2001; Baldwin 2002). Baldwin (2002) found that although other disciplines were each able to define what was unique about their role, there was no consensus as to what nurses brought by virtue of their nursing background. He concluded that there is a risk that if nurses cannot develop a clearer rationale for their role, or better articulate their unique contribution, that role might be lost.

Recent developments

Recent workforce policy threatens professional identity further through its focus on establishing more generic identities and new roles in mental health teams, including CAMHS. *New Ways of Working for Everyone* (DoH 2007) identifies 'creating capable teams' based on skills and competencies rather than the professional contributions that individual disciplines can bring to a multi-disciplinary team.

All personnel working with children and their families require an understanding of the assessment, detection, treatment and management of mental health problems in children (DoH 2004). Nurses work across a variety of settings and tiers in CAMHS (HAS 1995). They are involved in all of the above activities to varying degrees and are therefore in a position to influence the situation. Moreover, guidance for reform of the children's workforce emphasizes staff development across all disciplines, including the acquisition of common core skills and knowledge in order to achieve the five key outcomes of supporting children to be healthy, stay safe, enjoy and achieve, make a positive contribution and achieve economic well-being (DfES 2003, 2005; DoH 2004). Competencies associated with effective communication and engagement with children, young people, their families and carers, child and adolescent mental health development, safeguarding and promoting the welfare of the child, supporting transitions, multi-agency working and sharing information are all identified as important in the policies already referred to. With these changes CAMH nursing needs to focus on both art and science – i.e. evidence-based health care and interpersonal relationships.

Thus, the scope, impact and significance of the role played by CAMH nurses has developed, with nurses perceived as having an important role to play in the rapidly changing field of CAMH. Williams and Gale (2003) suggest that the future growth of nursing is essential for the success of initiatives to develop CAMHS in the early twenty-first century. However, the expansion of nursing roles in CAMHS can only be achieved successfully if nurses' continuing professional development needs are met. Nurses currently make up the largest professional group within CAMHS, therefore the need for nurses trained in the appropriate mental health skills is crucial. Yet the training of nurses is probably the least organized when compared to other CAMHS disciplines (Welsh National Assembly 2000). The majority of CAMH literature is not written specifically for nurses, and there appears to be a dearth of literature written by nurses in this field, with what there is coming mainly from North America. The creation of CAMH nurse consultant posts is viewed as an opportunity to tackle this issue as it enables highly skilled clinicians to remain in clinical practice (Williams and Gale 2003). Where evidence is lacking, nurse consultants contribute towards the development of the CAMH knowledge base by embarking on associated research activities (McDougall 2005).

The future of nursing in CAMHS

The Chief Nursing Officer (CNO) review of mental health nursing (DoH 2006) states that: 'pre-registration training programmes will prepare *all* mental health nurses to provide effective and values-based care' and that 'all pre-registration courses need to be reviewed' (p. 49). How this will be carried forward and nurses prepared for working in CAMHS remains to be seen. CAMH features little in pre-qualification nurse curricula. Pre-registration courses for mental health nurses are not designed to equip newly-qualified nurses to work in, or deal with, the mental health needs of children and young people (Jones 2004; DoH 2006). One explanation for this is that the client group falls between two different specialities – children's nursing and mental health nursing – and nurses working with this client group rarely receive relevant pre-registration training (Jones 2004). Thus, many feel that they lack the knowledge, skills and confidence to work effectively with the client group: as a result, specific and tailored post-registration education and training is needed (Jones 2004).

The CNO review identifies that all mental health nurses should continue to develop skills and knowledge throughout their careers (DoH 2006). Relating this to CAMH, postgraduate training plans which give nurses greater access to career opportunities and produce a partnership approach to education between universities and services are needed (Gale and Vostanis 2003). Unfortunately, many post-registration courses fail to prepare nurses for more extended roles in CAMHS, such as those which include consultation and multi-agency collaboration, and there-fore restrict nursing careers (Limerick and Baldwin 2000). Furthermore, there are few appropri-ate post-registered training programmes for CAMH nurses to equip them for these new roles (Jones 2004). The ENB 603 course no longer exists and there are now only a few centres in the country offering the equivalent of this course. Interestingly, evaluation of mental health nurses holding such qualifications highlights that only 34 per cent of 87 services employed nurses so qualified (Williams and Gale 2003). The University of Leicester is one centre that offers a comprehensive course in CAMH and it is in part through running this course that the need for this book came to be realized.

The contents of the book

We begin in Chapter 1, where mental health and illness are defined, before we look at the issue of stigma and its consequences. We also review some specific interventions undertaken with children and young people to manage stigma. This leads into Chapter 2 on child and family development. Child development is often very well described in psychology texts, but we considered a chapter highlighting key issues as essential – development is an aspect that no one working with children can ignore and Das Gupta and Frake offer a critique of the major theories. In Chapter 3 the aetiological factors associated with child mental health problems are presented and in Chapter 4, Leighton considers some of the legal and ethical issues that arise clinically for CAMH nurses. This is an excellent example of how the art and science touched on here come together in practice. These four chapters set the context for working as a nurse within SCAMHS. Chapter 5 covers assessment and highlights aspects such as culture and risk, which are increasingly on the agenda. Chapters 6 to 12 deal with the nature of the work undertaken by CAMH nurses. They include psychotherapeutic and counselling approaches, CBT, family work, nurse prescribing, working in inpatient units, multi-agency working and working with vulnerable children. In each of these chapters, our colleagues have taken the principles from specialist contexts that can be applied by any nurse working in CAMHS. The aim is to help nurses deliver the best care they can in whatever context they work. The authors have offered practical case examples and tried to evidence the work where such evidence is available. Unfortunately, as noted earlier, the evidence in some areas is relatively weak.

Chapter 13 covers clinical governance, audit and supervision, which are all key components of nursing roles. Again, there is relatively little available on how nurses fulfil these roles in practice. Chapter 14 provides an overview of different sources of CAMHS evidence. It addresses the role nurses play in research, highlighting some of the difficulties they face in developing such roles. Finally, in Chapter 15, the role of nurses in service development is reviewed. This chapter highlights the importance of nurses being involved in the activities discussed in Chapters 13 and 14, enabling them to fully contribute to service planning and delivery. Chapter 15 also explores the challenges ahead for nurses and indeed other professionals. Wider systematic changes within CAMHS provide an opportunity for CAMH nurses to demonstrate that nursing is both an art and a science. There is an emphasis on interdependent techniques and skills that are evidence based. These techniques and skills are applied within a therapeutic relationship, and are based on the identification of humanistic needs.

We hope you find this book helpful in your work. We remain convinced that nurses have an important contribution to make in providing CAMHS and we are committed to pledging our support and sharing our experience to contribute to their continuing professional development.

References

Baldwin, L. (2002) The nursing role in out-patient child and adolescent mental health services, *Journal of Clinical Nursing*, 11: 520–5.

Buchanan-Barker, P. and Barker, P. (2008) The tidal commitments: extending the value base of mental health recovery, *Journal of Psychiatric and Mental Health Nursing*, 15: 93–100.

Crow, R.A., Chase, J. and Lamond, D. (1995) The cognitive component of nursing assessment: an analysis, *Journal of Advanced Nursing*, 22: 206–12.

DfES (Department for Education and Skills) (2003) *Every Child Matters*. London: DfES.

DfES (Department for Education and Skills) (2005) *Common Core of Skills and Knowledge for the Children's Workforce*. London: DfES.

DoH (Department of Health) (2004) *National Service Framework for Children, Young People and Maternity Services*. London: DoH.

DoH (Department of Health) (2006) *From Values to Action: The Chief Nursing Officer's Review of Mental Health Nursing*, www.dh.gov.uk/en/Publicationsandstatistics/Publications/PublicationsPolicyAndGuidance/DH_4133839, accessed 21 April 2006.

DoH (Department of Health) (2007) *Mental Health: New Ways of Working for Everyone. Developing and Sustaining a Capable and Flexible Workforce. Progress Report*. London: DoH.

DoH (Department of Health) and DfCSF (Department for Children, Schools and Families) (2007) *A Profile of*

Child Health, Child and Adolescent Mental Health and Maternity Services in England 2007. Durham: University of Durham.

Gale, F. and Vostanis, P. (2003) The primary mental health worker within child and adolescent mental health services, *Clinical Child Psychology and Psychiatry*, 8(2): 227–40.

HAS (Health Advisory Service) (1995) *Child & Adolescent Mental Health Services*. London: HAS.

Heginbotham, C. and Williams, R. (2005) Achieving service development by implementing strategy, in R. Williams and M. Kerfoot (eds) *Child and Adolescent Mental Health Services: Strategy, Planning, Delivery, and Evaluation*. Oxford: Oxford University Press.

Jones, J. (2004) *The Post-Registration Education and Training Needs of Nurses Working With Children and Young People with Mental Health Problems in the UK*. London: RCN.

Leighton, S. (2008) Bereavement therapy with adolescents: facilitating a process of spiritual growth, *Journal of Child and Adolescent Psychiatric Nursing*, 21(1): 24–34.

Leighton, S., Smith, C., Minns, K. and Crawford, P. (2001) Specialist child and adolescent mental health nurses: a force to be reckoned with? *Mental Health Practice*, 5(2): 8–13.

Limerick, M. and Baldwin, L. (2000) Nursing in outpatient child and adolescent mental health, *Nursing Standard*, 15(13): 43–5.

McDougall, T. (2005) Child and adolescent mental health services in the UK: nurse consultants, *Journal of Child and Adolescent Psychiatric Nursing*, 18(2): 79–83.

Meltzer, H., Gatward, R., Goodman, R. and Ford, T. (2000) *Mental Health of Children and Adolescents in Great Britain*. London: TSO.

Norman, I. and Ryrie, I. (2005) Mental health nursing: origins and orientations, in I. Norman and I. Ryrie (eds) *The Art and Science of Mental Health Nursing*. Maidenhead: Open University Press.

Paterson, J.G. and Zderad, L. (1988) *Humanistic Nursing: The Phenomenological Theory*. New York: National League for Nursing.

Peplau, H. (1952) *Interpersonal Relations in Nursing*. New York: GP Putman.

Roper, N., Logan, W. and Tierney, A. (1986) Nursing models: a process of construction and refinement, in B. Kershaw and J. Salvage (eds) *Models for Nursing*. Chichester: Wiley.

Rosenbrock, H. (1987) Engineers and the work that people do, in R. Finnegan, G. Salaman and K. Thompson (eds) *Information Technology: Social Issues*. Milton Keynes: Open University Press.

Varcoe, C. (1996) Disparagement of the nursing process: the new dogma? *Journal of Advanced Nursing*, 23: 20–125.

Welsh National Assembly (2000) *Child and Adolescent Mental Health Services: Everybody's Business*. Cardiff: Welsh National Assembly.

Williams, R. and Gale, F. (2003) Current approaches to working with children and adolescents, in B. Hannigan and M. Coffey (eds) *The Handbook of Community Mental Health Nursing*. London: Routledge.

1 Defining mental health and mental illness

Sharon Leighton and Nisha Dogra

Key features
- Discussion of the terminological confusion that exists in relation to issues associated with mental health.
- The scale of individual suffering from mental health problems and illness among young people.
- The worldwide phenomenon of the stigmatization of mental illness, originating during childhood.
- Evidence regarding interventions to reduce stigma.

Introduction

In this chapter we explore the concepts of mental health and mental illness from different perspectives, including those relating to children, and of children. This is important as those who work in mental health, or are familiar with the field, often make the assumption that the terms used are readily understood by others. The scale of the problem and access to services is outlined. We then discuss stigma generally, explore the reasons for it and possible sequelae, and then consider how this relates to children. Finally, interventions to reduce stigma are briefly presented. As mentioned in the Introduction, where possible we have referred specifically to the literature relating to children but where this is limited we have drawn from the wider literature to highlight key issues.

The chapter begins with an exercise which provides a practical context for the theoretical content and should be borne in mind as you read, and answered once you have finished the chapter.

Box 1.1
Exercise
General questions

- What words or images do you associate with the following terms:

  - Mental health
  - Mental health problems
  - Mental illness
  - Mental disorder

- What sorts of problems do people experience that could be described as mental health problems or mental illness?
- How would you be able to tell if someone was experiencing mental health problems or mental illness?

Case scenarios and associated questions

Please read each senario and then consider the following questions in relation to it:

- What do you think might be happening with the young person?
- Do you think the young person has a mental health problem or illness? If so, on what grounds would you justify that decision?
- Do they need help?
- If so, who and/or what might be helpful?
- How might this be helpful?

Case scenario 1

Jack, aged 9, lives with his mother and younger brother. His father unexpectedly left the family a year ago. Jack started a new school six months ago and is having difficulty settling in. He complains of tummy ache each school morning and is increasingly reluctant to attend.

Case scenario 2

Emily, aged 14, lives with her parents, who are both busy professionals. She works hard, achieves A-grades and plans to be a lawyer. Recently she has been teased by her friends about her weight and has decided to go on a strict diet. She is pleased with the results so far and plans to continue eating little, making herself sick after meals and exercising a lot.

Case scenario 3

Joshua, aged 15, lives with his dad and stepmother. He has little contact with his mum or younger brother and sister. Recently he has been cautioned by the police for joy-riding in stolen cars with his mates. He prefers to spend time smoking dope with older boys rather than going to school.

Defining mental health and mental illness

Clarity is essential when using the terms 'mental health' and 'mental illness'. In all phases of a recent small-scale research project, conceptual confusion was identified in the literature review and among participants (Leighton 2008). Ironically, referring to mental illness in terms of mental health originated in the 1960s in an attempt to reduce stigma (Rowling *et al.* 2002). There is no widely agreed consensus on the meaning of these terms and their use. Mental health and mental illness can be perceived as two separate, yet related, issues.

Ryff and Singer (1998) suggest that health is not a medical concept associated with absence of illness, but rather a philosophical one that requires an explanation of a *good life* – being one where an individual has a sense of purpose, is engaged in quality relationships with others, and possesses self-respect and mastery. This is synonymous with the World Health Organization (WHO) (2000, 2005b) definition of positive mental health.

However, such a definition is incomplete as individuals do not exist in isolation, but are influenced by, and influence, their social and physical environments. Furthermore, people will have their own individual interpretations of what a *good life* is. Rowling *et al.* (2002: 13) define mental health as the capacity of individuals and groups to interact with one another and the environment in ways that promote subjective wellbeing, the optimal development and use of cognitive, affective and relational abilities, the achievement of individual and collective goals consistent with justice.

This is a more rounded definition, and one that can coexist alongside the WHO (1992) definition of mental disorder.

Mental health – one of many factors

It is also important to recognize that neither physical nor mental health exist separately – mental, physical and social functioning are interdependent (WHO 2004). Furthermore, all health issues need to be considered within a cultural and developmental context, as do the social constructs of childhood and adolescence (Walker 2005). The quality of a person's mental health is influenced by idiosyncratic factors and experiences, their family relationships and circumstances and the wider community in which they live (WHO 2004). Additionally, each culture influences people's understanding of, and attitudes towards, mental health issues. However, a culture-specific approach to understanding and improving mental health can be unhelpful if it assumes homogeneity within cultures and ignores individual differences (WHO 2004). Culture is only one, albeit important, factor that influences individuals' beliefs and actions (Tomlinson 2001; Dogra 2003). Interaction between different factors may lead to different outcomes for different individuals.

It can be argued that the above approaches are rooted in western perspectives. However, they provide a useful starting point from which to discuss mental health issues with children and their families.

Definitions of child mental health

Definitions of mental health as they relate specifically to children have been provided by the Health Advisory Service (HAS) (1995) and the Mental Health Foundation (1999). These definitions bear similarities to those provided by Ryff and Singer (1998) and Rowling et al. (2002), while recognizing the developmental context of childhood – i.e. the ability to develop psychologically, emotionally, creatively, intellectually and spiritually; initiate, develop and sustain mutually satisfying personal relationships; use and enjoy solitude; become aware of others and empathize with them; play and learn; develop a sense of right and wrong; and resolve problems and setbacks and learn from them (HAS 1995; Mental Health Foundation 1999). Such definitions are useful as they relate to 'societal' expectations of children.

Different definitions are used to define mental ill health. The WHO uses the term 'mental disorders' broadly, to include mental illness, intellectual disability, personality disorder, substance dependence and adjustment to adverse life events (WHO 1992). The WHO acknowledges that the word 'disorder' is used to avoid perceived greater difficulties associated with 'illness' – for example, stigma and the emphasis on a medical model. Meltzer et al. (2000) use the term 'mental disorders' in reference to emotional, conduct, hyperkinetic and less common disorders as defined by the ICD (International Classification of Diseases) 10 and DSM (Diagnostic and Statistical Manual of Mental Disorders) IV. Jorm (2000) focuses specifically on depression and psychosis. Meanwhile, Rowling et al. (2002) use the terms 'mental illness' and 'mental disorder' interchangeably. Johns (2002) and the British Medical Association (BMA 2006) identify that the term 'mental health problems' is used to cover a broad spectrum of conditions ranging from diagnosable disorders such as anxiety and depression, through to acting out behaviours. The BMA (2006) also distinguish between mental disorders and illness, with illness being severe psychiatric disorders such as depression and psychosis.

Others take a broader view. Rickwood *et al.* (2005) refer to 'young people's help-seeking for mental health problems' and proceed to use various terms including 'psychological distress', 'mental health issues', 'mental health problems' and 'mental disorder'. The interchangeable use of these terms in effect renders them meaningless, as their use may reflect an individual's bias, or political correctness, rather than indicating the extent or severity of the problem. However, all identify alterations in mood, thinking and behaviour associated with distress or impaired functioning across various domains.

Entity or dimension?

Kendall (1988) presents the relative merits of using categories and dimensions with respect to mental disorders. Typically, medicine has used categories, given its roots in the biological sciences. Categorization allows for easier definitions, recognition if someone fits a particular category and therefore conformity with a clinical concept. However, a dimensions approach allows for greater flexibility. Kendall (1988) concludes that where psychotic illness is concerned a categorical approach may be preferable, whereas in other conditions the situation is more likely to be changeable, and would perhaps benefit from a dimensional perspective.

One way of distinguishing between distress associated with adverse life events and more severe disorders which involve physiological symptoms and underlying biological changes is to distinguish between mental health problems and mental illness, using a multi-dimensional model. This has an additional advantage in enabling normal 'distress' (e.g. grief following bereavement) to be recognized as part of the 'human condition', rather than being medicalized and possibly classed as 'depression'. It is suggested that a variety of normal human experiences have become medicalized through an ever increasing range of psychological disorders with virtually every type of behaviour eligible for a medical label (e.g. social phobia, over-eating disorder, dependent personality disorder) (Illich 1977; WHO 1992; American Psychiatric Association 1994).

Rowling *et al.* (2002) propose that mental health and mental illness can be seen to exist as part of a multi-dimensional model. An exemplar of mental health and mental illness being two separate and yet related continua can be found in the vulnerability-stress working model developed by Asarnow *et al.* (2001). This model suggests how the effects of ongoing stress on mental health can lead to mental illness (depression) if left unchallenged.

Depression is classed as a diagnosable disorder which is reported to be on the increase (WHO 1996). However, the term 'depression' is also employed in everyday language for a variety of states of distress: demoralization as a result of long-term suffering; living with chronic adversity and stress; reaction to loss; low self-esteem; and pessimistic outlook. While there are similarities between the feelings of unhappiness, despondency, frustration and sense of hopelessness associated with a state of emotional stress and with depression, the latter involves pervasive physical symptoms such as sleep and appetite disturbance, and, ultimately, changes in brain chemistry. However, the cut-off between what is 'normal' stress and what is depression may not always be clear. It is not just the presence of symptoms that defines a disorder but also its severity and pervasiveness as well as its impact on everyday functioning.

Thus, from a dimensional perspective, many features of mental disorder (psychosis excepted) can be viewed as part of the range of 'normal' human behaviour. For example, anxiety is a normal human response to the perception of danger. Different types of anxiety are developmentally appropriate during childhood – for example, separation is an issue for infants, academic performance can cause anxiety during middle childhood and peer rejection concerns adolescents (Moore and Carr 2000).

Mental health literacy

Finally, in this section, it is also worth considering how the mental health 'literacy' of adults and children in the general population varies from that of professionals. In all phases of a recent research project, conceptual confusion was identified in the literature review and among adolescent participants (Leighton 2006, 2008). Focus group participants did not find the single continuum model suggested by the WHO (2000) helpful (Leighton 2006). Furthermore, in the focus group feedback session, participants suggested that labelling serious mental illnesses such as schizophrenia and major depression, as 'mental health problems', diminishes the seriousness of mental illness, with implications for attitudes towards, and treatment of, those with mental illness (Leighton 2006). It is also evident that there is considerable confusion for young people between the terms 'mental health', 'mental illness' and 'learning disability' (Dogra *et al.* 2007; Rose *et al.* 2007).

However, whatever terminology is used, the scale of individual suffering from mental health problems and illness is significant, and this is now briefly outlined.

The scale of the problem

The number of people experiencing mental health problems worldwide is reported to have risen to nearly epidemic proportions, with depression identified as the leading cause of disability among 15–44-year-olds (WHO 1996). In the UK the prevalence of mental health problems among adolescents is high. One in 20 is reported to be experiencing mental health problems at any given time (Mental Health Foundation 1999; Meltzer *et al.* 2000; Coleman and Schofield 2005). The Office for National Statistics (ONS) survey carried out in 1999 identified the following prevalence rates of diagnosable mental disorder among 11–15-year-olds: depression 1.8 per cent; anxiety 4.6 per cent; conduct disorder 6.2 per cent (Meltzer *et al.* 2000). Moreover, the prevalence of serious mental illness increases greatly during adolescence (Davidson and Manion 1996; Smith and Leon 2001; Rickwood *et al.* 2005). Such problems have a negative impact on an individual's development across all areas of their lives – i.e. self-esteem, relationships, academic success, career options and lifestyle (Mental Health Foundation 1999; Meltzer *et al.* 2000). Furthermore, the burden of adolescent mental health problems and illness involves enormous financial costs to individuals, families and society. These include loss of earnings for parents and adolescents, and social care, health service, education and Home Office costs (Appleton and Hammond-Rowley 2000). Although the scale of the problem is vast, studies indicate that less than a fifth of young people who need mental health care actually receive any services and, of those who do receive services, less than half obtain services appropriate to their need (Atkins *et al.* 2003; Hinshaw 2005).

Stigma and mental illness

In this section the aim is to explore the concepts of, and the relationship between, stigma and mental illness. One possible reason for both conceptual confusion and reluctance to seek help is that the stigmatization of mental illness continues to be a worldwide phenomenon (Jorm *et al.* 1997; Crisp *et al.* 2000; Sartorius 2002; Gureje *et al.* 2005).

Definition of the concept of stigma

Stigma can be viewed as a social construct. Setting people apart from other members of society has a long history. In ancient Greece members of tainted groups – for example, slaves and traitors – were branded with a mark (Goffman 1970; Hinshaw 2005). The concept is applied in diverse circumstances, including with reference to the mentally ill (Link and Phelan 2001). Additionally, stigmatization can be seen to depend on social, economic and political power and can occur on a large and tragic scale – for example, the systematic and dreadful stigmatization of the Jewish people by the Nazis (Link and Phelan 2001). Stigma was defined by Goffman (1970) as the position of the individual who is disqualified from full social acceptance. It is perceived as the outcome of a process of social labelling which singles out difference, names this difference inferiority, subsequently blames those who are different for their otherness and contributes to the creation of a spoilt identity (Goffman 1970). Since that seminal development, the concept has evolved. For example, stigma can be described with reference to the relationships between a set of interrelated concepts, rather than focusing solely on personal attributes – i.e. stigma exists when elements of labelling, stereotyping, separation, status loss and discrimination occur together in a power situation that allows these processes to happen (Link and Phelan 2001).

The nature and extent of stigmatization in adult mental illness

There are many factors involved in the formation of individuals' beliefs about mental illness, and their attitudes and behaviour towards those labelled as mentally ill. These include personal experience of mental illness, either personally or in someone known to them; the impact of the media; beliefs as to what causes mental illness (e.g. genetic, self-inflicted); and socio-cultural influences (Hinshaw 2005).

Four possible explanations for the stigmatization of mental illness have been identified in the research literature:

- dangerousness;
- attribution of responsibility;
- belief that mental illness is chronic with a poor prognosis;
- disruption of normal social interactions based on social rules (Hayward and Bright 1997).

These explanations can be elaborated as follows: people with mental illness are perceived as dangerous and unpredictable; there is an implied belief that the mentally ill choose to behave as they do and have only themselves to blame for their situation; people with mental illness are believed to respond poorly to treatment, and outcomes are poor, therefore they are an embarrassment and should be avoided; the mentally ill are seen as difficult to communicate with and this makes for unpredictable social intercourse. These are enduring themes, provoking personal fear in others and threatening to upset the status quo (Hayward and Bright 1997; Eminson 2004).

Explanations for the stigmatization of the mentally ill include the following ideas.

- From a biological perspective, a person suffering from mental illness may be viewed as a poor genetic choice in relation to reproductive potential and as a possible threat to the safety of the individual.
- The need to share understanding in order to survive as an individual and as a species means that when a person's way of perceiving the world is unfamiliar to us we can feel threatened and uncertain as to how to respond to them (Eminson 2004).

Media, mental illness and stigma

There is a dearth of research which focuses specifically on how mental illness is depicted in the children's and young persons' media (Wahl 2002). This is despite suggestions that such media provide the means by which young people will derive a preliminary understanding of mental illness. Participants in a small-scale local study identified some positive and accurate representations in the media. These included the Jacqueline Wilson books, the film *A Beautiful Mind* and Channel 4 documentaries (Leighton 2006). Byrne (2003) discusses examples in soap operas when television can perform a major public service where care is taken over how mental illness is portrayed. One suspects that the converse is also true – that when care is not taken the damage done to those suffering with mental illness can be immense.

Two large-scale literature reviews have suggested that the media can be regarded as an important influence on community attitudes towards mental illness. It is considered that there is a complex and circular relationship between mass media representation of mental illness and public understanding, with negative media images promoting negative attitudes and resultant media coverage feeding off an already negative public perception. It is also thought that negative images will have a greater effect on public attitudes than positive portrayals (Francis *et al.* 2001; Edney 2004). Work by Wahl (2003) suggests that this is equally applicable to children.

Consequences of stigma

Stigmatization of the mentally ill is understood to be prejudicial to them, injurious to all aspects of their treatment in mental health services and damaging to their role as members of society (Hinshaw 2005). Stigmatization leads to individual and social discrimination against the stigmatized person. Several authors identify that the discriminatory behaviour displayed can be hostile or avoidant and that it operates throughout personal and social relationships, pervading the home, workplace, local community, health and social welfare systems. This can result in increased feelings of shame, increased personal and social impairment and isolation, perpetuation and worsening of an illness, reluctance to access health care and infringement of human rights (Link and Phelan 2001; Crisp 2004; Hinshaw 2005).

Children, mental illness and stigma

There is also a scarcity of research examining the issue of stigma in relation to children and mental illness (Wahl 2002; Hinshaw 2005). As described previously, the high prevalence of mental health problems in young people and their reluctance to access specialist services gives cause for concern. The indications are that children develop negative attitudes towards those with mental illness early on (Gale 2007). Additionally, adolescents are the adults of the future and therefore their beliefs and attitudes regarding mental health and illness will affect service development, the quality of life of those experiencing mental health problems and the help-seeking behaviour of individuals (Armstrong *et al.* 2000; Hinshaw 2005).

Box 1.2 highlights themes identified from work which focused on adolescents, mental illness and stigma, albeit to varying degrees and using different methods.

Box 1.2 Themes associated with mental illness and stigma identified by adolescents

- Negative attitudes towards groups described as deviant – for example, the mentally ill – were apparent by kindergarten and increased with age (Weiss 1986, 1994; Wahl 2002).

- Words and phrases used to describe people with mental health problems or mental illness were largely derogatory, with the most common labels being 'retarded', 'psycho(path)', 'spastic', 'mental', 'crazy' and 'nutter' (Bailey 1999; Pinfold et al. 2003).
- The most frequently cited causes of mental illness were stress, genetics and bad childhood experiences (Bailey 1999).
- Young people with experience of mental health problems described being met with negative attitudes and reactions from other people, including professionals (Scottish Executive 2005).
- Although adolescents stigmatized peers with both physical and mental illness, they had a greater tendency to stigmatize those experiencing a mental illness (Sessa 2005a, 2005b).
- Adolescents presenting in school with either a physical or mental illness were likely to be socially excluded, itself a risk factor for developing mental health problems (Sessa 2005a, 2005b).
- Providing mental health education could lead to a positive change in reported attitudes in the short term, especially among females and those reporting personal contact with someone who had a mental illness (Pinfold et al. 2003).
- Although adolescents with less knowledge about mental health and illness had more negative attitudes towards mental illness, this did not influence the willingness to seek help for mental health problems as much as other factors – for example, level of psychological distress, number of barriers to overcome in order to access help, or adaptability (Sheffield et al. 2004).

From the sparse literature available, it would appear that adolescents' attitudes towards mental illness tend to be negative and stigmatizing. The need for education among the public, and adolescents in particular, in order to combat the stigma of mental illness is highlighted in the literature (Davidson and Manion 1996; Armstrong et al. 1998; Esters et al. 1998; Bailey 1999; Secker et al. 1999; Taylor 2001; Naylor et al. 2002; Pow 2003; Hinshaw 2005; Sessa 2005b).

Early indicators from our own work in Nigeria are that such attitudes transcend culture (Dogra 2009). However, there is evidence that stigma can be tackled. We will now examine some of the interventions undertaken to reduce stigma among children.

Interventions to reduce stigma

Large-scale interventions, such as high profile campaigns, are often difficult to evaluate. In the UK there have been several such campaigns – for example, The Royal College of Psychiatrists' campaign, 'Every Family in the Land' (Crisp 2004) and the WHO 'Dare to Care' campaign (WHO 2001). There is little evidence available to indicate that these have successfully changed public or personal attitudes, although there is evidence that more targeted initiatives may reap benefits (WHO 2005a). While much of the work to date has focused on adults, there are increasing efforts to address the issue among younger populations.

There is scope for joint working between schools and child and adolescent mental health services (CAMHS) in order to provide mental health promotion and reduce stigma. However, it is important that we do not attempt to reduce stigma by just changing the terminology used, as there is no evidence that such strategies work.

One small-scale local study found that young people thought they might be helped by having more basic information about local services (Dogra *et al.* 2007). In another such study, adolescents who lived with parental mental illness suggested that the best ways of providing adolescents with information about mental health included real experience and focusing on the issue in schools – i.e. existing sources of (mis)information. It was thought that those speaking out should be adolescents who were confident to talk about their situation, but they should not talk to people they knew for fear of being bullied and they should be pupils at other schools (Leighton 2006).

Two school-based interventions reported promising results. Rahman *et al.* (1998) concluded that the school programme they undertook was successful in improving mental health awareness in the children and their community. Unfortunately, the intervention is only briefly described and it is difficult to be clear whether attitudes towards mental health (and issues about stigma) were addressed, or whether awareness of mental health (and therefore knowledge and understanding) informed the intervention. More recently, Pinfold *et al.* (2003) undertook short educational workshops with 472 secondary school children in the UK. Changes were most marked for female students and those who had personal contact with people with mental health problems. Further analysis of the labels used to stigmatize people with mental illness found that of the 472 students sampled, 400 of them provided 250 words to describe a person with mental illness. Nearly half were derogatory (Rose *et al.* 2007). The authors conclude that there need to be interventions which address factual information about mental illness and that reduce the strong negative emotional reactions to people with mental illness. Effective evaluation is unlikely to be possible if there is no clarity about the purpose of the intervention or too many aspects covered in one evaluation (Naylor *et al.* 2002).

Summary

Considerable terminological confusion exists in relation to issues associated with mental health generally and among children and young people specifically. Furthermore, stigmatizing attitudes towards mental illness and related issues continue to pose a challenge. Children, young people and adults display similar negative attitudes towards both mental illness and individuals experiencing mental health problems or illness. However, there is some evidence that these might be amenable to interventions such as education.

You may now wish to reflect on the issues discussed in this chapter by returning to the exercise in Box 1.1.

References

American Psychiatric Association (1994) *Diagnostic and Statistical Manual of Mental Disorders*, 4th edn. Arlington, VA: American Psychiatric Association.

Appleton, P.L. and Hammond-Rowley, S. (2000) Addressing the population burden of child and adolescent mental health problems: a primary care model, *Child Psychology and Psychiatry Review*, 5(1): 9–16.

Armstrong, C., Hill, M. and Secker, J. (1998) *Listening to Children*. London: The Mental Health Foundation.

Armstrong, C., Hill, M. and Secker, J. (2000) Young people's perceptions of mental health, *Children and Society*, 14: 60–72.

Asarnow, J.R., Jaycox, L.H. and Thompson, M.C. (2001) Depression in youth: psychosocial interventions, *Journal of Clinical Child Psychology*, 30(1): 33–47.

Atkins, M.S., Frazier, S.L., Adil, J.A. and Talbot, E. (2003) School based mental health services in urban communities, in M.D. Weist, S.W. Evans and N.A. Lever (eds) *Handbook of School Mental Health: Advancing Practice and Research*. Hingham, MA: Kluwer Academic/Plenum Publishers.

Bailey, S. (1999) Young people, mental health and stigmatization, *Psychiatric Bulletin*, 23: 107–10.

BMA (British Medical Association) (2006) *Child and Adolescent Mental Health: A Guide for Health Care*

Professionals, www.bma.org.uk/ap.nsf/AttachmentsByTitle/PDFChildAdolescentMentalHealth/$FILE/ ChildAdolescentMentalHealth.pdf, accessed 5 August 2007.

Byrne, P. (2003) Psychiatry and the media, *Advances in Psychiatric Treatment,* 9: 135–43.

Coleman, J. and Schofield, J. (2005) *Key Data on Adolescence,* 5th edn. Brighton: Trust for the Study of Adolescence.

Crisp, A. (2004) The nature of stigmatisation, in A.H. Crisp (ed.) *Every Family in the Land: Understanding Prejudice and Discrimination against People with Mental Illness.* London: Royal Society of Medicine Press.

Crisp, A.H., Gelder, M., Rix, S., Meltzer, H.I. and Rowlands, O.J. (2000) Stigmatisation of people with mental illnesses, *British Journal of Psychiatry,* 177: 4–7.

Davidson, S., and Manion, I.G. (1996) Facing the challenge: mental health and illness in Canadian youth, *Psychology, Health and Medicine,* 1(1): 41–55.

Dogra, N. (2003) Cultural competence or cultural sensibility? A comparison of two ideal type models to teach cultural diversity to medical students, *International Journal of Medicine,* 5(4): 223–31.

Dogra, N. (2009) *Training School Counsellors and Young People in Secondary Schools in Ibadan, Nigeria on Common Mental Health Problems with an Emphasis on Tackling Stigma,* project report for the British Council. Leicester: University of Leicester.

Dogra, N., Vostanis, P., Abuateya, H. and Jewson, N. (2007) Children's mental health services and ethnic diversity: Gujarati families' perspectives of service provision for mental health problems, *Transcultural Psychiatry* 44(2): 275–91.

Edney, D.R. (2004) *Mass Media and Mental Illness: A Literature Review,* www.ontario.cmha.ca/content/ about_mental_illness/mass_media.asp?fontaction=plus, accessed 14 Januray 2005.

Eminson, M. (2004) Personal responses to a lack of shared perception, in A.H. Crisp (ed.) *Every Family in the Land: Understanding Prejudice and Discrimination against People with Mental Illness.* London: Royal Society of Medicine Press.

Esters, I.G., Cooker, P.G. and Ittenbach, R.F. (1998) Effects of a unit of instruction in mental health on rural adolescents' conceptions of mental illness and attitudes about seeking help, *Adolescence,* 33(130): 469–76.

Francis, C., Pirkis, J., Dunt, D. and Blood, R.W. (2001) *Mental Health and Illness in the Media: A Review of the Literature,* http://ausinet.flinders.edu.au/resources/other/mhimedia.pdf, accessed 14 Januray 2005.

Gale, F. (2007) Tackling the stigma of mental health in vulnerable children and young people, in P. Vostanis (ed.) *Mental Health Interventions and Services for Vulnerable Children and Young People.* London: Jessica Kingsley.

Goffman, E. (1970) *Stigma: Notes on the Management of a Spoiled Identity.* New York: Penguin.

Gureje, O., Lasebikan, V.O., Ephraim-Oluwanuga, O., Olley, B.O. and Kola, L. (2005) Community study of knowledge of and attitude to mental illness in Nigeria, *The British Journal of Psychiatry,* 186: 436–41.

HAS (Health Advisory Service) (1995) *Child & Adolescent Mental Health Services.* London: HAS.

Haywood, P. and Bright, J.A. (1997) Stigma and mental illness: a review and critique, *Journal of Mental Health,* 6(4): 345–54.

Hinshaw, S.P. (2005) The stigmatisation of mental illness in children and parents: developmental issues, family concerns and research needs, *Journal of Child Psychology and Psychiatry,* 46(7): 714–34.

Illich, I. (1977) *Disabling Professions.* New York: MarionBoyars Publishers.

Johns, S. (2002) Young people, schools and mental health services: intervention or prevention? in L. Rowling, G. Martin and L. Walker (eds) *Mental Health Promotion and Young People: Concepts and Practice.* Roseville, NSW: McGraw-Hill Australia.

Jorm, A.F. (2000) Mental health literacy: public knowledge and beliefs about mental disorders, *British Journal of Psychiatry,* 177: 396–401.

Jorm, A.F., Korten, A.E., Jacomb, P.A., Christenson, H., Rodgers, B. and Pllitt, P. (1997) 'Mental health literacy': a survey of the public's ability to recognize mental disorders and their beliefs about the effectiveness of treatment, *Medical Journal of Australia,* 166: 182–6.

Kendall, R. (1988) Diagnosis and classification, in R. Kendall and A. Zealley (eds) *Companion to Psychiatric Studies.* Edinburgh: Churchill Livingstone.

Leighton, S. (2006) Pilot thesis: 'What do I think? Where do I go?' Exploring adolescents' understanding of mental health issues and their attitudes towards seeking help for mental health problems. Unpublished doctoral assignment.

Leighton, S. (2008) 'What do I think? Where do I go?' Exploring adolescents' understanding of mental health issues and their attitudes towards seeking help for mental health problems. Unpublished doctoral thesis.

Link, B.G. and Phelan, J.C. (2001) Conceptualising stigma, *Annual Review of Sociology*, 27: 363–85.

Meltzer, H., Gatward, R., Goodman, R. and Ford, T. (2000) *The Mental Health of Children and Adolescents in Great Britain*. London: The Stationery Office.

Mental Health Foundation (1999) *Bright Futures: Promoting Children and Young People's Mental Health*. London: Mental Health Foundation.

Moore, M. and Carr, A. (2000) Anxiety disorders, in A. Carr (ed.) (2000) *What Works with Children and Adolescents?* London: Routledge.

Naylor, P., Cowie, H., Talamelli, L. and Dawkins, J. (2002) *The Development of Adolescent Pupils' Knowledge about and Attitudes Towards Mental Health Difficulties*, project report to PPP Healthcare Medical Trust, www.ukobservatory.com/projects/project3.html, accessed 9 January 2005.

Pinfold, V., Toulmin, H., Thornicroft, G., Huxley, P., Farmer, P. and Graham, T. (2003) Reducing psychiatric stigma and discrimination: evaluation of educational interventions in UK secondary schools, *British Journal of Psychiatry*, 182: 342–6.

Pow, J. (2003) A study of adolescents in Fife (15–16 years) to establish their views, attitudes and knowledge of mental health issues, unpublished MSc dissertation, University of Dundee.

Rahman, A., Mubbashar, M.H., Gater, R. and Goldberg, D. (1998) Randomised trial of impact of school mental health programme in rural Rawalpindi, Pakistan, *The Lancet*, 352: 1022–5.

Rickwood, D., Deane, F.P., Wilson, C.J. and Ciarrochi, J. (2005) Young people's help-seeking for mental health problems, *Australian e-Journal for the Advancement of Mental Health*, 4: supplement, www.ausinet.com/journal/vol4iss3suppl/rickwood.pdf, accessed 5 August 2007.

Rose, D., Thornicroft, G., Pinfold, V. and Kassam, A. (2007) 250 labels used to stigmatise people with mental health, *BMC Health Services Research*, 7: 97.

Rowling, L., Martin, G. and Walker, L. (eds) (2002) *Mental Health Promotion and Young People: Concepts and Practice*. Roseville, NSW: McGraw-Hill Australia.

Ryff, C.D. and Singer, B. (1998) The contours of positive human health, *Psychological Inquiry* 9(1): 1–28.

Sartorius, N. (2002) Iatrogenic stigma of mental illness, *British Medical Journal*, 324: 1470–1.

Scottish Executive (2005) *See Me . . . Let's Stop the Stigma of Mental Ill Health*, www.seemescotland.org, accessed 25 May 2005.

Secker, J., Armstrong, C. and Hill, M. (1999) Young people's understanding of mental mealth, *Health Education Research*, 14(6): 729–39.

Sessa, B. (2005a) I'll have to lie about where I've been, *Young Minds Magazine*, 76: 34–5.

Sessa, B. (2005b) Comparing adolescents' opinions towards mental and physical illness: a stigma survey, personal correspondence, 18 May 2005.

Sheffield, J.K., Fiorenza, E. and Sofronoff, K. (2004) Adolescents' willingness to seek psychological help: promoting and preventing factors, *Journal of Youth and Adolescence*, 33(6): 495–507.

Smith, K. and Leon, L. (2001) *Turned Upside Down: Developing Community-based Crisis Services for 16–25 Year Olds Experiencing a Mental Health Crisis*, London: Mental Health Foundation.

Taylor, C. (2001) Adolescent perceptions of mental health services and of mental health, unpublished BSc thesis, University of Leicester.

Tomlinson, M. (2001) A critical look at cultural diversity and infant health synergy, *Australian Transcultural Mental Health Network*, winter: 3–5.

Wahl, O.F. (2002) Children's views of mental illness: a review of the literature, *Psychiatric Rehabilitation Skills*, 6(2): 134–58.

Wahl, O.F. (2003) Depictions of mental illnesses in children's media, *Journal of Mental Health*, 12: 248–58.

Walker, S. (2005) *Culturally Competent Therapy: Working with Children and Young People*. Basingstoke: Palgrave Macmillan.

Weiss, M.F. (1986) Children's attitudes towards the mentally ill: a developmental analysis, *Psychological Reports*, 58: 11–20.

Weiss, M.F. (1994) Children's attitudes towards the mentally ill: an eight-year longitudinal follow-up, *Psychological Reports*, 74: 51–6.

WHO (World Health Organization) (1992) *International Statistical Classification of Diseases and Related Health Problems*, 10th revision. Geneva: WHO.

WHO (World Health Organization) (1996) *The Global Burden of Disease*. Geneva: WHO.

WHO (World Health Organization) (2000) *World Mental Health Day. Mental Health: Stop Exclusion – Dare to Care*, http://who.int/world-health-day/en/, accessed 2 December 2005.

WHO (World Health Organization (2001) *World Mental Health Day. Mental Health: Stop Exclusion – Dare to Care*, http://www.emro.who.int/MNH/WHD/WHD-Brochure.pdf, accessed 2 July 2009.

WHO (World Health Organization) (2004) *Promoting Mental Health: Concepts, Emerging Evidence, Practice: Summary Report*. Geneva: WHO.

WHO (World Health Organization) (2005a) *Child and Adolescent Mental Health Policies and Plans*. Geneva: WHO.

WHO (World Health Organization) (2005b) *WHO European Ministerial Conference on Mental Health: Facing the Challenges, Building Solutions: Stigma and Discrimination Against the Mentally Ill in Europe*, http://www.euro.who.int/document/MNH/ebrief10.pdf, accessed 12 July 2008.

2 Child and family development

Mani Das Gupta and Clay Frake

> **Key features**
> - Exploration of theories relating to cognitive development.
> - Overview of socio-emotional development.
> - Discussion of family development as a context for child development.

Introduction

This chapter focuses on general aspects of the cognitive and socio-emotional development of children as well as family development, with the aim of providing a broad overview of key ideas in these areas. First, different theories of cognitive and emotional development are discussed. This is followed by a section on the family, focusing on the importance of understanding the family context when dealing with child development.

The development of the child

There are five universally recognized stages of childhood (prenatal, infancy, toddlerhood, childhood and adolescence), although these stages may have different names in different cultures (Whiting and Edwards 1988). Children also go through stages of development in at least five different domains: neural, physical, social, emotional and cognitive.

Theories of cognitive development

Studying cognitive development involves looking at *cognition*, the act or faculty of knowing (including logical reasoning, problem-solving and concept formation) that underlies the process of change in both cognitive and social development.

There are a number of theories of cognitive development. This chapter starts with Piaget's (1992) classic theory because it is the most comprehensive to date and has significantly influenced current theory and research.

Piaget's stage theory of development

Piaget revolutionized the study of children's cognitive development by proposing that infants and children *construct* their own knowledge, and that they learn and think in *qualitatively* different ways from each other and from adults. Piaget's proposal was radically different from the behaviourist view that regarded the child as passively shaped by external forces.

According to Piaget, intelligent behaviour is one aspect of a general biological tendency towards *adaptation* and *organization*. Any adaptation to the environment necessarily implies an organization within the individual – they are seen as parallel processes. Just as the body has physical structures that help it adapt to the environment, Piaget believed that the mind also builds *psychological structures* (organized ways of making sense of experience) or *schema*, that enable organization and adaptation.

Organization is the internal rearrangement and linking together of schemes to form an interconnected cognitive system. For instance, initially infants can suck and grasp, but they cannot coordinate these actions. After a while they can both grasp and suck an object. According to Piaget, a higher level of organization has occurred – two basic schemes (grasping and sucking) have been combined – indicating adaptation to the environment.

Adaptation involves building schemes through direct interaction with the environment. Two complementary processes explain how schemes are formed and developed:

- *assimilation* (the external world is interpreted in terms of current schemes);
- *accommodation* (old schemes are adjusted and new ones created to produce a better fit with the environment).

These processes work together. When children are not changing very much they assimilate more than they accommodate, a state Piaget refers to as *cognitive equilibrium*. However, during times of swift cognitive change (when new information does not match current schemes) and they switch from assimilation to accommodation, children are in a state of *disequilibrium* (cognitive discomfort). Once schemes have been modified children shift back to assimilation, using new structures until they need to be modified again. Piaget called this back and forth process *equilibration* – the individual moves towards *cognitive equilibrium*. Each time equilibration occurs, more effective schemes are produced. Piaget used the processes of *organization, adaptation* (assimilation and accommodation) and *equilibrium* to explain how cognitive change occurs as children develop.

Development progresses by gradual (step by step) elaboration and extension of schemas according to Piaget. He proposed four major, universal, stages of development. In addition to universality, stages are characterized by qualitatively different cognitive structures (and modes of reasoning). Each stage has specific sub-stages. Each stage is not only derived from the previous stage (incorporating and transforming it) but also follows an invariant sequence. That is, Stage 1 always comes before Stage 2; regression is not possible. Children's thinking differs from stage to stage in a steady progression towards logical reasoning (Harris and Butterworth 2002).[1] Each stage is now discussed.

Sensory-motor stage (0–2 years)

In the *sensory-motor stage* infants progress from reflexive actions and focusing on sensory and motor experiences to being capable of forming representations and beginning to think. Innate reflexes (e.g. sucking) are accommodated to particular parts of the body and other objects (e.g. thumb, cloth). Babies move through the various sub-stages until they reach the last sub-stage called *internal representation*. An example Piaget gave of the child acquiring internal representation was that of *deferred imitation* when the child copies a behaviour that he or she has seen before, but which is not currently present. In the first two years of life the infant develops from reflexive responding to active exploration of the world, using symbolic representation.

---

[1] For a simple description of each stage and more on Piaget's background go to http://psychology.about.com/od/ piagetstheory/a/keyconcepts.htm or http://findarticles.com/p/articles/mi_g2699/is_0004/ai_2699000417.

Pre-operational stage (2–6/7 years)

During the *pre-operational stage* there are tremendous strides in language. Piaget acknowledged language as the most flexible form of representation but believed that thought and language developed separately. Thought is not only independent of language, it is a sensory motor activity that occurs before language, leading to representations of experience which children then label using words.

A key limitation to the child's thinking during the pre-operational period is *egocentrism* – the inability to distinguish other people's viewpoints from one's own. Egocentrism may lead young children to attribute their own thoughts and feelings to other people, and even to inanimate objects. Piaget called this tendency *animism*. Another characteristic of the pre-operational stage is *centration* – centring or focusing on a single aspect of a problem and ignoring other aspects. Centration is demonstrated most clearly in Piaget's *conservation* experiments.

Conservation involves understanding that certain physical characteristics of objects remain the same even when their appearance changes. Children are shown two identical objects (or sets of objects) and one of these is changed. The child is then asked if the objects are still the same. Typically, a pre-operational child finds it hard to understand that if an object is changed in shape or appearance (e.g. a ball of clay is rolled into a sausage shape) its qualities (e.g. quantity, volume) remain the same (it's the same amount of clay; children typically say the sausage shape has more clay in it). Piaget argued that the child focuses or centres on one dimension (shape) and does not *compensate* for the change in the other dimension (amount). Furthermore, Piaget said that the child cannot understand the notion of *reversibility* – the sausage can be rolled back into a ball.

Concrete operational stage (6/7–11/12 years)

During the *concrete operational stage* thought is logical, flexible and organized, but still tied to concrete information. Children are no longer egocentric and also pass standard conservation tasks. Nevertheless, according to Piaget, the capacity for *abstract reasoning* is still lacking. For instance, given the question 'Edith is fairer than Susan. Edith is darker than Lily. Who is the darkest?', concrete operational children become confused, but given dolls (concrete objects) to rank in order they solve the problem easily. During this stage children also demonstrate *seriation* – the ability to arrange items along a quantitative dimension such as length or weight. They are able to seriate mentally (*transitive inference*) as well as have mental maps of large scale environments (*cognitive mapping*). Despite this, Piaget argues that they are tied to using concrete objects to think logically.

Formal operational stage (11/12 years onwards)

In the final *formal operational stage* children move beyond their concrete experiences and begin to think in abstract and logical ways. During this stage adolescents are able to represent and manipulate thought processes in three ways, which they were unable to do previously. They become:

- able to combine ideas logically and use deductive reasoning to find explanations for problems;
- systematic problem-solvers through using scientific reasoning;
- able to think about possibilities rather than just reality; to think abstractly, and to consider the consequences of their actions, making long-term planning possible.

Hypothetico-deductive reasoning, a key characteristic of this stage, is the ability to reason hypothetically. When faced with a problem, adolescents start with a *general theory* of all the possible factors that might affect an outcome and *deduce* specific *hypotheses* or *predictions* about what might happen. Then they *test* these hypotheses in an orderly fashion to see which one will work in the real world (e.g. performance on Piaget's pendulum problem).[2]

Critiques of Piaget's work

Piaget's work has been criticized for a number of reasons, including the fact that stages are not universal – children attain the stages at different times in different cultures (Dasen 1972; Harris and Butterworth 2002). Schooling also improves results on Piagetian tasks (Harris and Butterworth 2002). Another criticism is that the formal operation stage is often not attained until much later on, if at all, even in western cultures (Girotto and Light 1992; Cole *et al.* 2001). Finally, the tasks themselves have been criticized as not making 'human sense' to the child (Donaldson 1984). Children may make mistakes because they misread the experimenter's intentions, for example, or because they are unfamiliar with the task material. Children's understanding and use of language can also interfere with performance on these tasks (Donaldson 1986).

One of Donaldson's main criticisms of Piaget's theory was that tasks did not make sense to children and therefore underestimated their level of thought. McGarrigle and Donaldson (1975) found that pre-schoolers could succeed at a conservation of number task if the cause of the transformation made more sense to the child (for instance, if a 'naughty teddy' was responsible for the transformation rather than the experimenter). Donaldson argued that children get it wrong in the Piagetian form of the task because they try to make sense of what the adult experimenter is doing, and for children to succeed the task needs to make *human sense* not just logical sense. Similarly, asking the question twice makes the child think that their answer to the first question must have been wrong, so they give a different answer when the question is repeated (Samuel and Bryant 1984). In terms of egocentrism, it has been found that pre-schoolers can adapt their speech to fit the needs of listeners – 4-year-olds use shorter, simpler sentences when talking to 2-year-olds than to age-mates (Shatz and Gelman 1973). Children's failures on classic Piagetian tasks indicate their reasoning is not as well developed as that of children in the next stage.

Despite these criticisms, when tests are done exactly as Piaget did them, the findings are the same. It is worth noting that many of Piaget's ideas have influenced modern thought about cognitive development. The most useful contribution may be that children's thinking changes radically from stage to stage, and it is unreasonable to expect a 4-year-old to be able to reason like a 10-year-old.

Another major criticism concerns the formal operational stage. Many adolescents and adults do not become formal operational thinkers at all; only about a third develop formal operational thought, while others may only show formal operational thought in their area of expertise (e.g. a physicist may show abstract reasoning in his field while not being able to appreciate abstract poetry).

Piaget suggested that enormous changes in children's thinking occur in the pre-school and school years. Children's vocabulary expands and they learn the conventions of language and conversation. Around the age of 6, children begin to understand 'operations' or concepts such as addition, multiple classification, reversibility and the use of inductive logic. Recent research on this period confirms that huge changes in thinking do take place that are not tied to Piaget's ages and stages (Siegler 1991; Harris and Butterworth 2002). Siegler's work, for instance, shows

---

[2] See http://www.springerlink.com/content/k101m060123522m4/.

that cognitive development is not as step-wise as Piaget suggested. Children are more likely to use a variety of strategies, of varying complexity, in solving a problem. There is an age-related change as strategies become more complex with age.

Vygotsky's theory of cognitive development

Piaget saw the development of logical understanding as running parallel with the development of social understanding, and believed that development in these two areas could be studied independently of each other. Vygotsky (1896–1934) was one of the first to criticize this idea. Whereas Piaget believed that cognitive development was a spontaneous process and that cognitive structures develop without any direct teaching from adults, Vygotsky[3] (1986) argued that teaching and direct instruction by adults was crucial to cognitive development, and emphasized the *cultural context* of development.

There is evidence that children do benefit from both social interaction and direct instruction (Wood *et al.* 1976; Ginsburg-Block *et al.* 2006). There is also evidence that, in a number of areas, children internally modify existing schemes (e.g. the object concept or drawing; language is perhaps one of the best examples of this). According to Vygotsky, social and intellectual development cannot be studied independent of each other as social understanding holds the key to intellectual development. Vygotsky defined intelligence as *the capacity to learn from instruction* and saw the teacher's role as central to development. He believed that the teacher (or knowledgeable other) should extend and challenge the child to go beyond their current level of competence (Harris and Butterworth 2002). Both Piaget and Vygotsky agreed that development occurs in stages and that active participation by the child is essential for learning.

For Vygotsky, two levels of development occur simultaneously:

- Level 1: the actual, 'present level of development' – i.e. what a child can do on their own;
- Level 2: the 'potential level of development' – i.e. what a child can do in collaboration with adults.

Vygotsky called the gap between the actual and potential levels of development the *zone of proximal* (or next) *development* (ZPD). The ZPD indicates what the child is ready to master next, given the best possible adult support, on the basis of present achievements. Children learn through direct instruction from more knowledgeable people around them. This 'expert intervention', Vygotsky argued, should be at a level beyond their current thinking, but not so far ahead that the instruction is beyond their comprehension (i.e. within their ZPD).

One of Vygotsky's main contributions was his emphasis on the role of teaching. For Vygotsky, the *teaching-learning* process is a *social exchange* and *shared meanings* are built up through joint activity. The word 'teaching' usually refers to schooling, but formal teaching was not what Vygotsky had in mind. He used 'teaching' in a much broader sense to cover situations in which a more knowledgeable other (parent, adult, or more experienced peer) works with a child, with the aim of guiding the child's behaviour and improving the child's competence. This is more of an 'apprenticeship' model (Rogoff 1990). Children learn to do a task not just by watching and copying an adult, but through the adult's direct interventions, which help to *scaffold* the child's learning (Wood *et al.* 1976).

Both Piaget's and Vygotsky's ideas have been supported as well as challenged by more recent research. Despite the criticisms that can be made of their work, both men revolutionized the way in which psychologists and others view children's cognitive processes and capabilities.

---

[3] Online resources at http://www.kolar.org/vygotsky/.

Information processing approaches to cognitive development

There is no single information processing (IP) theory of development but all these approaches focus on the flow of information through the cognitive system and how individuals *process* information. IP approaches liken human thinking to a complex *storage, retrieval and organizing* system for information, similar to a computer. Individuals manipulate information, monitor it, and then organize it. The brain is seen as being analogous with the computer's hardware, and cognitive activities with its software. Although these comparisons are not perfect, this analogy has contributed to developing a view of the *mind as an active information processing system*. Changes in hardware are compared to changes in the brain (e.g. myelination) while changes in software are likened to the acquisition of new strategies (e.g. memory strategies).

Typically IP approaches do not describe individuals as being at one stage or another, in the Piagetian sense, focusing instead on the precise, detailed steps involved in mental activities. The focus is on how information is stored, retrieved, organized and manipulated. As information is processed gradually, the amount of information that can be processed at each step is limited. With brain development, children's information processing *capacity* increases enabling more efficient processing. Development is seen as a continuous process, as illustrated in Figure 2.1. Limitation on cognitive capacity is overcome as long-term memory capacity increases, behaviour becomes *routinized* and *strategies* are developed to link input more effectively with output.

The acquisition of knowledge, through experience, as well as the development of memory capacity, is very important in IP theories. Older children and adults have more *accumulated knowledge* so can process information more rapidly and use more effective problem-solving strategies. As more information becomes available in long-term memory this is rapidly applied to new problems, leading to improved competence (Siegler 1991).

Unlike IP theorists, developmental psychologists are more interested in the *emergence* of

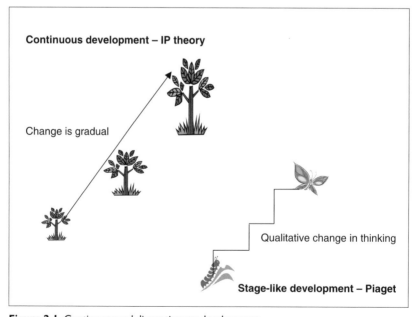

Figure 2.1 Continuous and discontinuous development

knowledge. Dreyfus and Dreyfus (1986) proposed a five step sequence of development from *novice* to *expert*. The differences between these steps lie in:

* experience;
* commitment to the problem (increasing with expertise);
* the degree to which knowledge has been automated;
* awareness of theory behind knowledge.

IP theorists argue that the speed and efficiency of the cognitive system improves with age and experience. One form of this efficiency is the greater use of different types of *processing strategies* with age, associated with memory development. Pre-school children use some memory strategies, but they do not do so consistently. School-age children on the other hand use such strategies much more consistently and more often.

Integrating Piaget and IP theory

Case (1992) integrated Piagetian and IP approaches and proposed that increases in available capacity (rather than an equilibration process) was the major mechanism for development. Total memory capacity is fixed, but available capacity increases as strategy use becomes automatic. With practice, many skills become more automatic and automatic activities require less effort and little use of capacity. Improved efficiency means less memory capacity is used and is due to both

* biological maturation of the brain; and
* increased automation of activities.

For Case and other neo-Piagetians, the major change underlying development is not change in logic, but change in the *amount* of information a child can handle at any one time. Children's successes with logical problems are an offshoot of their increasing information processing ability. One major difference between the information processing approach and Piaget's theory is that in the former development is continuous, whereas Piaget believed that thinking is qualitatively different at different stages.

Emotional development

The emotional development of the child begins very early. It has been argued that babies are born with the ability to interact, and though the interaction may initially be regulated by an adult, infants gradually begin to instigate, as well as direct, social interchanges (Schaffer 1996). In a cross-cultural study involving Chinese, Canadian and North American babies, Kisilevsky *et al.* (1998) asked the mothers to adopt a still face, unreactive pose or depressed emotional state. When infants tried to get their parent to respond. lack of parental reaction led to infants turning away, crying and frowning. Identical results across cultures suggest that there is a built-in withdrawal response to parental lack of communication.

Social interaction

Social interaction in infancy is important and not only for attachment. Lack of positive interactions between infants and caregivers can lead to other negative long-term outcomes for the child. In a longitudinal study of maternal mental health, Caplan *et al.* (1989) interviewed 92 women and their first-born children. Children of mothers who were depressed had more behavioural difficulties. Additionally, marital disharmony during pregnancy and paternal psychiatric problems were associated with later childhood behaviour problems. Murray and Cooper's (1999) review of the effects of post-partum depression on infants indicates that in the long term these infants may be at risk of breakdown when facing stress, as well as behavioural and cognitive problems.

Understanding emotion

By school age, children can refer to causes, consequences and behavioural signs of emotions and use social referencing to direct their own behaviour. They know that unpleasant events cause anger/sadness. By the age of 6 or 7, children understand mixed feelings; they understand that people can experience two (contradictory) emotions at the same time (feel good and bad). The ability to see multiple, differing emotions is characteristic of the concrete operational stage. Emotional understanding develops through:

- interpreting emotions (social referencing);
- socialization;
- social experience – talking about feelings with parents and other adults;
- cognitive development;
- language (allows new ways of expressing and regulating feelings).

Figure 2.2 summarizes some of the key stages in emotional development (based on Bukato and Daehler 1998), outlining rough ages when children can be expected to develop the ability to display and deal with particular emotions. Primary emotions (happiness, sadness, fear) appear early and may be innate, but the child's *social* experiences shape and direct emotional behaviour to conform to *cultural norms*. The *self-conscious emotions* (shame, pride, guilt) appear

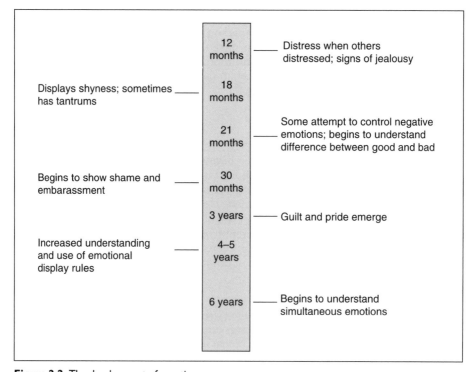

Figure 2.2 The development of emotions

at the end of the second year (with the emergence of a sense of self) and require both self-awareness and adult instruction.

Social referencing involves using another person's emotional reaction to understand a situation. By the age of 1, the principal caregiver's emotional expression (happy, angry, fearful) influences babies' reaction to strangers and new toys (Schaffer 1996). Social referencing eventually allows toddlers to compare their own reactions with those of others.

Culture and emotional expression

Culture affects emotional expression (Harris 1989) and influences the way children *express, manage* and *talk about* emotions. Emotional socialization is best illustrated in the cross-cultural study of display rules – rules that specify when, where and how it is culturally acceptable to display/express emotion by:

- setting limits to emotional expression;
- encouraging the expression of specific emotions;
- providing culture-specific norms for displaying emotions.

Display rules specify when, where and how it is culturally acceptable to display emotion. In one study comparing Japanese and North American children, researchers found that the Japanese control emotional display from nursery years; sharing is encouraged, crying is discouraged and overt displays of negative emotion (anger or jealousy) are unacceptable, and suppressed. Urban American mothers, on the other hand, encourage toddlers to display anger and aggression in 'self-defence' – for example, protecting a toy from another child (Harris 1989).

During early childhood children also develop the ability to recognize when someone is masking feelings. This ability seems to be universal but there are wide cultural variations in the ages at which children learn about masking emotions and the conditions when this is expected. Gender differences in ability to recognize and display masked emotions have also been identified, with girls recognizing and displaying masked emotions better than boys (Harris 1989).

Emotional regulation

Emotional reactions and the ability to regulate these reactions depend on children's interpretation of social contexts, understanding of display rules, and how well they understand the emotions and intentions of others. Socialization and parental control have a huge impact on this and affect *emotional regulation* (see Figure 2.3). Emotional regulation refers to the ability to modulate negative feelings.

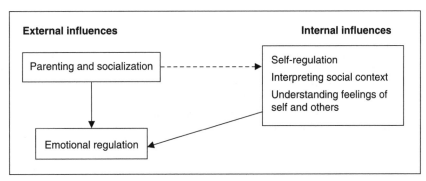

Figure 2.3 Influences on emotional regulation

Not all children learn to regulate their emotions. Inadequate emotional regulation can lead to social and adjustment problems such as:

- more frequent conflict with peers;
- less satisfying peer relationships;
- poor school adjustment (Eisenberg and Morris 2002; Lengua and Kovacs 2005).

Pro-social behaviour such as sharing, helping, caregiving and compassion (Grusec *et al.* 2002) is learnt through *explicit modelling* by adults, as well as by adults explaining what acceptable behaviour is and why children should behave in a pro-social manner. This is called 'emotional socialization' (you may recognize Vygotsky's approach here). Socio-emotional competence is the ability to behave appropriately when strong emotions are aroused (Saarni 2000), and requires:

- awareness of own emotional state;
- awareness of emotional state of others;
- capacity for empathy and sympathy.

The inability to understand the emotional state, goals and behaviour of self and of others is a major influence on aggression (Halberstadt *et al.* 2001). Denham *et al.* (2003) reported on a longitudinal study of 127 children using puppets to assess emotional knowledge. They asked the children what the puppet looked like in three different situations:

- basic (when sad);
- specific (after a nightmare);
- requiring *emotional masking* (when teased, but if she shows it she will get teased more).

Children chose a face (from a selection showing various expressions) and attached it to the puppet. Anger and antisocial behaviour were assessed through naturalistic observation and teacher reports. Denham *et al.* found that boys and girls who had less knowledge of emotions and expression in pre-school were more likely to be aggressive to peers later on. Children who understand the causes of emotion and how emotion is expressed are much less likely to behave aggressively (Lemerise and Arsenio 2000).

Aggressive children misinterpret social interactions and negative interpretation can lead to inappropriate aggressive responses. Berkowitz (2003) suggests that aggression also results from negative feelings in frustrating situations. When a child 'fails' to win approval or achieve a goal, the negative emotions that arise initiate a *flight-or-fight* response. Although the tendency to withdraw or become aggressive is linked to primitive emotions of fear or anger, these initial feelings can be significantly modified by cognitive processes. For instance, if a child is playing with a toy which a playmate snatches, the child may experience negative feelings, and depending on temperament and past social experiences, may want to react aggressively. If the child has internalized a 'no-hitting' rule, and knows that violating that rule has certain consequences, they may instead ask for help from a teacher or parent.

Cognitive and emotional development both play important, connected, roles in the development of the child. Through cognition children learn to think and reason about the world around them. By learning to understand and regulate emotions, children integrate into their social worlds. Both these aspects are required for appropriate social development. However, no child develops in a vacuum, and the next section looks at one of the most important contexts of child development – the family.

Family development

In this section we only consider family development, as working with families is considered in more detail in Chapter 7. Family development is examined within a family therapy context. The difficulty in applying this model in practice is then discussed before briefly reviewing early theories on family development used by family therapists and how these ideas have evolved. As described earlier, child development is relatively well understood and has a sound evidence base and universal application (with some cross-cultural caution).

A pragmatic definition of what a family is would include everybody who is involved in meeting a child's immediate emotional and developmental needs. This could include parents and their partners, siblings, grandparents and close friends (Dogra *et al.* 2009). It is important to be guided by the family's definition, so as not to impose your own values on clients.

Family therapy grew out of the ideas developed by systems theorists in the 1940s and 1950s. The family was regarded as a system which had a range of self-regulating mechanisms governing its functioning, which in turn can be observed and influenced if necessary. The notion therefore that the family system would have a life cycle and hence its own developmental pathway was a natural extension of this theory, with attempts to define developmental milestones and common patterns through observation of families. Building upon existing ideas of individual life cycles, Haley (1973) described the family life cycle one might expect the 'typical' family to experience and the transitional challenges to its integrity it might have to face. This was expanded upon and developed as a therapeutic tool by Carter and McGoldrick (1989) and became a highly influential model in the field of family therapy (see below). This model remains a useful aid when working with families to help them develop an understanding of their current dilemmas. The model proposed separate stages of family life through which a family passes during its development.

Stages of the family life cycle

- Family of origin experiences.
- Leaving home.
- Pre-marriage stage.
- Childless couple stage.
- Family with young children.
- Family with adolescents.
- Launching children.
- Later life.

The points of *transition* between these stages were recognized as potentially difficult times for families and their ability to manage would be influenced by family patterns, beliefs, circumstances at the time and wider societal influences. As family therapy theory was developed, particularly by feminist therapists, it became clear that what were attempts to be descriptive about families easily became prescriptive and families who did not fit into a 'normal' pattern could be viewed as pathological or dysfunctional. Dallos and Draper (2000: 54) commented that 'in one sense the concept of the family life cycle merely maps a formal set of assumptions that people in a given society hold about a particular form of family life'.

The family life cycle model was based on an idealized, white, western, heterosexual family ideal, with mother, father and several children in an intact family. This does not reflect real life as experienced by many people. For instance, step-families with children from previous relationships and children from the current relationship may be at different life cycle stages simultaneously. Practice based on this model can easily become oppressive as it reflects dominant societal discourses and potentially disqualifies the choices individuals and families make about how to conduct their lives.

A family's development is shaped by wider contextual factors (culture, ethnicity, class, gender, sexuality) as well as by their history, intergenerational patterns of behaviour and communication. An example of this is the difference between cultures regarding what are considered appropriate levels of intimacy, closeness and levels of dependency.

Box 2.1 **Exercise**	• How might a family's handling of an adolescent's passage into independence be influenced by each of wider contextual factors such as culture, ethnicity, class, gender, sexuality and family-specific factors such as family history, intergenerational patterns of behaviour and communication? • How was this transitional stage in family development managed in your own family?

If the notion of a single unifying template of family development seems impractical and undesirable, how can the concept of family development be useful in child and adolescent mental health (CAMH) nursing? The family, irrespective of who forms it, remains the single most important context or system in which a child develops. An understanding of how that system itself develops can lead to more effective and appropriate interventions. The principle of development remains central, but being mindful of the family's unique circumstances and their view of the developmental challenges they face is also vital. This includes considering how a family is changing through developmental stages which may be inevitable, through the passage of time, or required of the family by events, such as divorce, migration and ill health. There may be some common concerns and themes with which all families have to contend. Gorrel-Barnes (1998: 47) described these as nurture, the organization of authority and power, and inter-dependence versus autonomy. Focusing on these themes with families, and listening to how they have been trying to manage and negotiate the changes as their family has developed contextualizes a child's individual development and mental health problems. It is also likely to provide possibilities for intervention and change.

Box 2.2 Exercise: case scenario

Tom is 16 and has a diagnosis of an autistic spectrum disorder and a mild learning disability. He has been referred to child and adolescent mental health services (CAMHS) with anxiety and low mood. His parents have been separated for several years. Tom lives with his mother who has chronic physical health problems and he sees his father every weekend. Tom will be leaving school soon and the plan is for him to start at college. Tom's parents both recognize that he is likely to need continuing support as he moves into adulthood, but they disagree on the nature and extent of that support. Tom's father feels he needs to be pushed to realize his potential and hopefully live semi-independently. His father's expectations often cause Tom considerable anxiety. His mother would prefer him to continue to live with her as they have a close relationship and Tom is very settled. However, this comfortable existence leads to increasing isolation and Tom becomes withdrawn and is reluctant to go out of the house. The tension between Tom's parents on this issue also makes Tom anxious. Tom's father comes from a white British working-class family who place a high value on hard work and self-reliance. His mother's parents moved to the UK from southern Europe 50 years ago, and she is part of a large extended family that enjoys frequent contact and high levels of mutual support.

- What family developmental issues can you identify?
- What normative assumptions are likely to be made by agencies about Tom and his family?

Families clearly experience a range of changes and challenges which could be framed as developmental, but these cannot be placed in a normative framework as each family is unique in its make-up, cultural background, history and beliefs about itself. The family has to adjust to each development of its members or transition, and difficulties in this adjustment process are often reflected in the mental health of young people.

Summary

Cognitive and emotional development does not occur in a vacuum – they are both influenced by social context, especially the family context. Understanding the family processes that impact on development is vital for effective intervention. In this chapter we have considered both child and family development, which are important to understanding children and child mental health. By engaging families in discussion about family development one might be able to help them better understand the issues they are facing. Clearly, child and family development are linked, although they have been considered separately for ease of discussing key aspects.

References

Berkowitz, L. (2003) Affect, aggression, and antisocial behaviour, in R.J. Davidson, K.R. Scherer and H.H. Goldsmith (eds) *Handbook of Affective Sciences*. New York: Oxford University Press.

Bukato, D. and Daehler, M.W. (1998) *Child Development: A Thematic Approach*. New York: Houghton Mifflin.

Caplan, H.L., Cogill, S.R., Alexandra, H., Robson, K.M., Katz, R. and Kumar, R. (1989) Maternal depression and the emotional development of the child, *British Journal of Psychiatry*, 154: 818–22.

Carter, E.A. and McGoldrick, M. (1989) *The Changing Family Life Cycle. A Framework for Family Therapy*, 2nd edn. New York: Gardner.

Case, R. (1992) *The Mind's Staircase*. Hillsdale, NJ: Erlbaum.

Cole, M., Cole, S. and Lightfoot, C. (2001) *The Development of Children*. New York: Worth.

Dallos, R. and Draper, R. (2000) *An Introduction to Family Therapy: Systemic Theory and Practice*. Buckingham: Open University Press.

Dasen, P.R. (1972) Cross-cultural Piagetian research: a summary, *Journal of Cross-Cultural Psychology*, 3: 2.

Denham, S.A., Blair, K.A., De Mulder, E., Levitas, J. and Sawyer, K. (2003) Preschool emotional competence: pathway to social competence? *Child Development*, 74(1): 238–56.

Dogra, N., Parkin, A., Gale, F. and Frake, C. (2009) *A Multidisciplinary Handbook of Child and Adolescent Mental Health for Front-line Professionals*, 2nd edn. London: Jessica Kingsley.

Donaldson, M. (1984) *Children's Minds*. London: Fontana.

Donaldson, M. (1986) *Children's Explanations: A Psycholinguistic Study*. Cambridge: Cambridge University Press.

Dreyfus, H.L. and Dreyfus, S.E. (1986) Mind over machine, *Journal of Personality and Social Psychology*, 32: 805–21.

Eisenberg, N. And Morris, A.S. (2002) Children's emotion-related regulation, *Advances in Child Development and Behaviour*, 30: 189–229.

Ginsburg-Block, M.D., Rohrbeck, C.A. and Fantuzzo, J.W. (2006) A meta-analytic review of social self-concept and behavioural outcomes of peer assisted learning, *Journal of Educational Psychology*, 98: 732–49.

Girotto, V. and Light, P. (1992) The pragmatic bases of children's reasoning, in P. Light and G.E. Butterworth (eds) *Context and Cognition*. Hemel Hempstead: Harvester.

Gorrel-Barnes, G. (1998) *Family Therapy in Changing Times*. Basingstoke: Palgrave.

Grusec, J.E., Davidov, M. and Lundel, L. (2002) Prosocial and helping behaviour, in P. Smith and C. Hart (eds) *Blackwell Handbook of Childhood Social Development*. Oxford: Blackwell.

Halberstadt, A.G., Denham, S.A. and Dunsmore, J.C. (2001) Affective social competence, *Review of Social Development*, 10(1): 79–119.

Haley, J. (1973) *Uncommon Therapy: The Psychiatric Techniques of Milton H. Erikson*. New York: W.W. Norton.

Harris, M. and Butterworth, G. (2002) *Developmental Psychology: A Student's Handbook*. Hove: Psychology Press.

Harris, P.L. (1989) *Children and Emotion*. Oxford: Blackwell.

Kisilevsky, B.S., Hains, S.M.J., Lee, K., Muir, D.W., Xu, F., Fu, G., Zhao, Z.Y. and Yang, R.L. (1998) The still-face effect in Chinese and Canadian 3–6 month old infants, *Developmental Psychology*, 34: 629–39.

Lemerise, E. and Arsenio, W. (2000) An integrated model of emotion processes and cognition in social information processing, *Child Development*, 71: 107–18.

Lengua, L. and Kovacs, E. (2005) Bidirectional associations between temperament and parenting and the prediction of adjustment problems in middle childhood, *Journal of Applied Developmental Psychology*, 26: 21–38.

McGarrigle, J. and Donaldson, M. (1975) Conservation accidents, *Cognition*, 3: 341–50.

Murray, L. and Cooper, P.J. (eds) (1999) *Postpartum Depression and Child Development*. New York: Guilford Press.

Piaget, J. (1992) *The Origins of Intelligence in Children*. Madison, CT: International Universities Press.

Rogoff, B. (1990) *Apprenticeship in Thinking*. Oxford: Oxford University Press.

Saarni, C. (2000) Emotional competence: a developmental perspective, in R. Bar-On and J. Parker (eds) *The Handbook of Emotional Intelligence*. San Francisco: Jossey-Bass.

Samuel, J. and Bryant, P. (1984) Asking only one question in the conservation experiment, *Journal of Child Psychology and Psychiatry*, 25: 315–18.

Schaffer, H.R. (1996) *Social Development*. Oxford: Blackwell.

Shatz, M. and Gelman, R. (1973) The development of communicative skills: modifications in the speech of young children as a function of listener, *Monographs of Society for Research in Child Development*, 38(5): 1–38.

Siegler, R.S. (1991) *Children's Thinking*, 2nd edn. Englewood Cliffs, NJ: Prentice Hall.

Vygotsky, L.S. (1986) *Thought and Language*. Cambridge, MA: MIT Press.

Whiting, B.B. and Edwards, C.P. (1988) *Children of Different Worlds: The Formation of Social Behaviour*. Cambridge, MA: Harvard University Press.

Wood, D., Bruner, J.S. and Ross, G. (1976) The role of tutoring in problem solving, *Journal of Child Psychology and Psychiatry*, 17: 89–100.

3 The aetiology of child mental health problems

Nisha Dogra, Mani Das Gupta and
Sharon Leighton

Key features
- Discussion of the multi-faceted nature of risk, which involves biological, psychological and environmental factors.

- Discussion of how risk involves factors within the child and their interplay with environmental factors.

Introduction

Risk factors for mental health problems among children can be broadly divided into biological, psychological or environmental, or any combination of these. However, although their mode of interaction remains unclear, risk factors rarely act in isolation (Surgeon General's Office 2009). Single aetiological factors (whether they be biological, psychological or social) may play a major role or quite a minor one, dependent on the disorder and the context. Sometimes factors may not be relevant in the causation of problems or disorders, but may be influential in maintaining a problem (e.g. a young person may become anxious following a particular event and the anxiety is then maintained because of family dynamics, and/or how the family manages the initial anxiety). Very often it is the interplay between the different factors that leads to development of problems.

In this chapter we outline each of these in turn, starting with individual risk factors before presenting a framework for thinking about specific environmental factors (the family and school peer relationships), and finally considering the wider socio-political context. The interaction between genetics and the wider environment is also highlighted. It is important to have an understanding of the aetiological factors that may play a part in the development of problems because some may be amenable to change, which will be relevant when it comes to treatment; some factors will be more easily managed or changed than others. We will not cover aetiological factors relating to specific disorders, except as examples to illustrate specific points. We would also highlight that the factors that protect against mental health problems (i.e. resilience) are often the opposite of those that cause such problems.

The chapter begins with an exercise in order to provide a practical context for the theoretical content.

Box 3.1
Exercise
- Before you read on, consider the last child or young person that you saw.
- What might be the possible risk factors for mental health problems?
- What, if any, are the social, the psychological or biological factors?

- Can you differentiate between factors that are causing the problem and those that maintain it?
- Discuss your findings with a colleague and see how much agreement there is between you.

Individual risk factors

Some of the risk factors inherent in the child are identified in Box 3.2.

Box 3.2 Risk factors in the child

- Low IQ and learning disability.
- Specific developmental delay.
- Communication difficulty.
- Difficult temperament.
- Physical illness, especially chronic, and/or neurological.
- Academic failure.
- Low self-esteem.

Temperament

Individual temperament may make some children more vulnerable than others. Even children who have the same level of vulnerability may not experience the same environments or risks; so some, who are predisposed, go on to develop problems while others do not. It is impossible to change a child's basic temperament but therapeutic interventions can help children in both managing those aspects of their temperament that may cause problems and in reinforcing their strengths.

There are three broad categories of temperament: difficult/feisty; anxious/slow to warm up; easy (Chess and Thomas 1999). Children with positive temperamental features are more likely to interact positively with others. The warm responses evoked enhance self-esteem and self-efficacy. Interactions between adults and children who both have difficult temperaments often result in disruptive behaviour, especially where there is family conflict. Regardless of levels of family conflict, children with difficult temperaments are more likely to show disruptive behaviour.

Specific temperamental traits pose a risk for the development of symptoms of anxiety and depression in children. High levels of factors reflecting negative affectivity (i.e. the degree of dissatisfaction with life and associated feelings of distress) appear to place children at risk for both disorders. Low levels of factors associated with positive affectivity (i.e. the level of pleasurable engagement in life and the extent to which a child feels enthusiastic and involved) appear to represent a specific risk for the development of depressive symptomatology (Lonigan *et al.* 2003).

Generally, children with lower cognitive levels are at increased risk of antisocial behaviour. Research suggests that lower IQ is a risk factor because such children have less problem-solving skills and are more vulnerable to family adversity (Koenen *et al.* 2009).

Style of attachment relationship

Attachment refers to a specific type of biologically based relationship, which provides a secure base from which children can explore the world (Bowlby 1969). Attachment relationships can be classified as either secure or insecure, with three types (ambivalent, avoidant or disorganized) of insecure relationship identified (Prior and Glaser 2006). Attachment behaviour is operational from birth, designed to ensure survival by stimulating *care-giving behaviour* from a parent/carer. It is subsequently triggered by separation, or threatened separation, from the attachment figure. Repeated experience of interactions and quality of care received result in the construction of an *internal working model* (IWM) of relationships from which generalized expectations are made. The manner in which the individual might predict and relate to the world, and approach other relationships, is determined by these IWMs (Bowlby 1969). Insecure attachment relationships, coupled with high levels of parental anxiety, are associated with increased risk of anxiety disorders in children (Manassis 2001).

Gender

There are a number of theories of gender development. *Social learning* theory proposes that children learn gender stereotypical roles through observation and imitation of the same-sex parent. *Cognitive development* theories argue that children actively construct gender identity (based on their experience of both genders). However, it is difficult to separate what comes from within the child and what is socially constructed. It is also difficult to separate gender from cultural contexts. Dwairy (2004) found that parents in Palestine and Egypt used different parenting styles for girls and boys in different contexts (Dwairy and Menshar 2006). Clinical experience tends to find that girls are more likely to present with emotional disorders (and self-harm, after adolescence) and boys with behavioural problems. It is unclear whether social expectations or genetics make girls more likely to internalize their problems and boys to express distress through externalizing behaviours. Boys have a higher prevalence rate for most neuro-developmental disorders such as autistic spectrum disorder (ASD) (Green et al. 2005). Eating disorders are generally much more common in girls (Pawluck and Gorey 1998).

Biological factors

Genetic factors are more important in some disorders such as attention deficit hyperactivity disorder (ADHD) and autistic spectrum disorder (ASD). The fact that children with learning disabilities are at increased risk of ADHD, ASD and other mental health problems indicates that biological factors may be more at play in this group than perhaps with others (Koenen et al. 2009). Box 3.3 highlights some of the biological factors that may impact on the development of mental health problems.

Familial factors are difficult to separate from genetic factors, as families may share the same genetic predisposition, to be anxious for example, while also sharing the same environment and thus learning patterns of behaviour.

Box 3.3 Biological factors that may be relevant in the development of behaviours that may be, or may mimic, mental health problems

- Trauma that affects the brain (e.g. road traffic accident, fall, abuse).
- Infection (e.g. meningitis).
- Tumours (e.g. meningioma).
- Chromosomal abnormalities (e.g. Down's syndrome, where there is an extra copy of chromosome 21; Klinefelter's syndrome, where boys have an extra X chromosome).

- Endocrine disorders (e.g. hypothyroidism may mimic depression; hyperthyroidism may mimic anxiety).
- Medical disorders, especially neurological problems and any chronic illnesses (e.g. cystic fibrosis).
- Toxicity (e.g. substance misuse, medication side-effects).

Environmental risk factors

Bronfenbrenner's (1979) model of layered contexts is fairly widely used. The contexts include the microsystem, mesosystem, exosystem and the macrosystem. The first layer (microsystem) includes the relationships that the child is actively involved in, for example, with parents, siblings and peers. These interactions depend on context and child characteristics. The meso-system describes how the different components of the microsystem come together. The exosystem is the wider local community such as the neighbourhood. The macrosystem is usually remote from any specific child, but may still be a major social influence, for example, socio-economic policy regarding child-rearing, education and health policies and the wider cultural and political contexts. It is worth noting that the influence of different factors may vary depending on the stage of the child's life. For example, some adverse family factors may be mitigated by external factors in older children. We will now take each of the major areas in turn, starting with the family.

The family

Box 3.4 Risk factors in the family

- Overt parental conflict.
- Family breakdown.
- Inconsistent or unclear discipline.
- Hostile or rejecting relationships.
- Failure to adapt to a child's changing needs.
- Physical, sexual and/or emotional abuse.
- Parental psychiatric illness.
- Parental criminality, alcoholism or personality disorder.
- Death and loss, including loss of friendship.

The family is usually the context in which children spend their early years, and is therefore a significant factor in the development of mental health problems. The family may be a risk factor in that children from large families are at greater risk, as are children from poorer families (Surgeon General's Office 2009). Nevertheless, healthy development is possible within a number of different family structures. Research on non-traditional families shows healthy development in a variety of family types (Schaffer 1998). Eiduson et al. (1999) measured a wide variety of behaviour in children from four different family structures (single-parent families, unmarried couples, families living in communes, traditional nuclear families). There were no significant differences across groups, indicating that the structure of a family may be less relevant than how it meets the needs of the children within it. One of the major influences of the family is through parenting.

Parenting styles

Parenting can be classified on a number of dimensions, including warmth, sensitivity, directiveness and punitiveness (Schaffer 1996). Baumrind (1966) identified two dimensions of parenting – demanding and responsive. Combinations of these led to the identification of three styles of parenting – authoritative, authoritarian and permissive (*laissez faire*). A fourth style, 'neglectful', was later added (Macoby and Martin 1983) – see Figure 3.1. The styles and child characteristics associated with each are described briefly below (based on Schaffer 1996).

Authoritative parents are high in control and responsiveness, valuing compliance and setting behavioural standards, while respecting the child's developing autonomy and independence. They expect developmental and age appropriate behaviour. Children of authoritative parents are the most competent, being more self-reliant, content, socially responsible, self-controlled and cooperative.

Authoritarian parents are low on responsiveness and high on demand/control. They set standards of behaviour demanding unrealistic levels of maturity. Obedience is valued and the child's autonomy and independence restricted. Punitive measures of control are preferred. Children tend to be surly, defiant, dependent and socially incompetent (especially boys).

Permissive parents are high on responsiveness, but low on control, tolerating more immature behaviour than other styles. They do not set consistent standards for the child's behaviour.

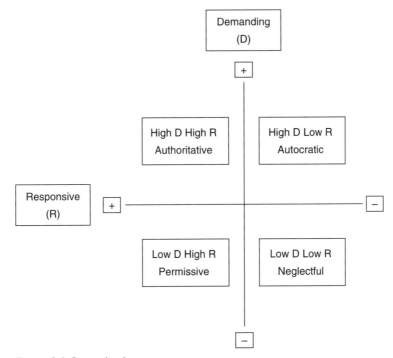

Figure 3.1 Parental styles

Children are more likely to be aimless, lacking in self-assertiveness, and generally non-achievement oriented.

Permissive neglectful parents provide no real care or supervision. There is little response by parents to children's needs (emotional or otherwise) and little is demanded of children, resulting in young people who may not have any behavioural boundaries (Macoby and Martin 1983).

Relationships within the family

The relationship between parental control and child outcome described above is a linear one – i.e. a certain style of parenting seems to lead to a certain outcome. However, there are a number of criticisms of this linear model (Das Gupta 1995). Firstly, children's behaviour both influences, and is influenced by, parental behaviour. Secondly, children's behaviour both influences, and is influenced by, parental relationships, which in turn impact on parenting behaviour (see Figure 3.2, based on Belsky and Vondra 1989). Parents influence children's behaviour, while each child's temperament and behaviour directly influences parental behaviour and parenting style. Every child is unique, so no two children are brought up by the 'same' parents.

A host of other factors affect relationships within the family (e.g. poverty, bereavement, divorce). Relationships within the family are also diverse and complex. Not only does a child have a unique relationship with each parent, they also have inimitable relationships with siblings, grandparents and other members of the extended family.

Dunn (1988: 119) emphasizes the importance of sibling relationships for social and emotional development, characterizing them as 'distinctive in emotional power and intimacy, qualities of competitiveness, ambivalence and of emotional understanding'. Sibling relationships are also important because they are often the most long-lasting of relationships, as most children outlive their parents. Siblings usually spend more time with each other than they do with either parent, and dealing with sibling rivalry and conflict are major parental concerns.

Sanders (2004) looked at whether sibling relationships compensate for, or are similar to, parent–child relationships. The *compensatory model* proposes that siblings may supply the needs that parents fail to meet (e.g. attachment, care, social interaction, stimulation). According to the *congruence model* parents provide models for social relationships; positive interactions between parents and between parents and children promote positive sibling relationships. Sanders concluded that research supports both models.

Dunn (1988) highlighted the importance of individual differences between children, as well as the child's age, in the study of sibling relationships. Siblings may have different interests at different ages, and rivalry at one stage can change to friendship at another, so longitudinal studies and monitoring of relationships is essential. In very difficult circumstances children may adopt strategies to simply survive by focusing solely on their own needs, which may

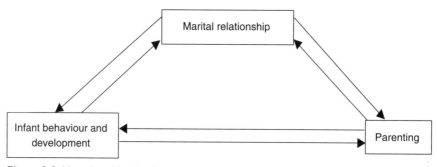

Figure 3.2 Mutuality of family influences

lead to negative consequences (competition and conflict). Thus, sibling relationships could be a crucial consideration within a multi-factorial aetiology approach to mental health problems.

Abuse

Abuse within the family context can lead to a number of problems. In younger children it may be expressed as behavioural problems. Early experiences of physical, sexual abuse and/or parental neglect are risk factors for depression and suicidal behaviour in adolescents (Brodsky and Stanley 2008).

Parental illness

Parental illness impacts directly on family dynamics and parental styles. A parent who is ill may be inconsistent in their parental style. Additionally, children may have to take on more family responsibilities. Children who are carers have different social, emotional and psychological needs than children of healthy parents and can often feel isolated and lonely. It may be difficult for these children to form stable peer relationships as they have less time to 'hang around' and are not able to go out as much as other children.

There is strong evidence that any parental illness, and especially mental illness, may have a significant impact on children's mental health (Manning and Gregoire 2006). Postnatally depressed mothers have problems in responding appropriately to the infant's behaviour, and typically show a lessening or lack of contingent responses to their infant's emotional signals. The effect is that the parent becomes less responsive to the child, there is less positive interaction and more inconsistent discipline (either lax or over-forceful). The effect on the child is that generally infants are more likely to be withdrawn, cry, display lack of energy and irritability and have attachment difficulties. Customary emotions tend to be negative (sadness or anger) rather than positive (joy or interest) (Pickens and Field 1993). Emotional development is affected, whereby children withdraw into a depressive mood to avoid parental insensitivity. Such children are more likely to develop behavioural problems and are more likely to mimic their parents' anger and become impulsive and antisocial. Cooper and Murray (1997) concluded that postpartum depression had a significant adverse impact on the family, especially on the dependent infant. It is of great concern that follow-up studies of the children of mothers who have experienced postpartum depression reveal an enduring adverse impact on the child's socio-emotional development. However, Cooper and Murray found some ameliorating effects. They suggested that treatment is successful in most cases of postnatal depression, and that a warm relationship with the father or other significant adult has a beneficial effect. They also suggest that a reduction of stressors (e.g. poor marital relationship, social support, financial difficulties) accompanying the depression can help.

The wider social environment

The focus here is on schools and peer relationships. Wider cultural and political contexts are then considered.

Box 3.5 Risk factors in the community

- Socio-economic disadvantage.
- Homelessness.

- Disaster.
- Discrimination.
- Other significant life events.

Schools

The school environment

Children spend a great deal of time in schools and the school environment can significantly impact on their mental health. It has long been established that there are certain types of schools that are associated with fewer mental health problems. Over the last decade there has been an increasing political emphasis on giving British schools responsibility for mental health promotion (DfES 2003). There has also been a significant amount of investment in promoting mental health in schools. The impact of such interventions has yet to be seen.

Schools can have a very positive impact on children and mitigate some of the negative impact of other social factors, providing a sense of belonging and security which may be lacking at home (Mortimore 1995). However, for some young people school is a considerable source of stress, worry and unhappiness, either because the demands of the academic work or peer relationships become too challenging. Unidentified learning difficulties may lead to behavioural problems for some young people and hence referral to mental health services. For others, unidentified mental health problems (such as ADHD) may mean that children fail to meet the expectations placed on them. Transition between junior and senior schools may also prove a considerable stressor as senior schools require children to be more independent.

It is evident that *mentally healthy* children are more likely to succeed in school, and that schools will be most successful in their educational mission when they promote academic, social and emotional learning (Elias *et al.* 1997). As Zins *et al.* (2004: 3) state, 'intrinsically schools are social places and learning is a social process so it comes as no surprise that schools can help young people develop self esteem and learn the language to acknowledge and address emotions' (both positive and negative). When asked what made young people feel good about themselves, a common response was 'doing well in school' (Gordon and Grant 1997). Conversely, not achieving in school has a negative impact on mental health.

Johnson and Johnson's (2004) framework demonstrates how schools can promote social and emotional learning through creating a cooperative community and promoting constructive conflict resolution and civic values. A cooperative community is effectively created where there is:

- a strong sense of positive interdependence;
- individual accountability for roles;
- promotion of each other's success;
- development of interpersonal and small group skills.

Successful schools not only have an internal sense of community, they also develop partnership with the families of young people and the wider community (Johnson and Johnson 2004). However, society as a whole may challenge these communal aspirations, as individuals, not communities, are judged for jobs and rewards. In addition, although teachers may state that they frequently recognize mental health needs among pupils and would welcome training, in practice this is not usually borne out (Gordon and Grant 1997).

It is worth considering bullying in the context of whole-school approaches. Clinically it is evident that the impact of bullying is intensified when children and/or their parents feel that the school has not taken the issue seriously. Since December 1999 all schools in the UK must have an anti-bullying policy by law, as stated in the School Standards and Framework Act 1998, Section 61(4b). However, as with many politically driven initiatives, although the paperwork may demonstrate the existence of such policies, the experience of children tells a different story. Bullying has immediate and longer-term effects. The immediate effects may be anxiety and school avoidance, although children may resist disclosure. Others may become withdrawn and their academic performance may deteriorate. Bond *et al.* (2001) found that bullying was associated with later anxiety and depression, especially for girls. Bullying can lead to children feeling marginalized and affect their self-esteem and confidence. In extreme cases it can lead to suicide.

Peer relationships

Peer acceptance is associated with a greater sense of belonging and fewer behavioural problems, and friendships alleviate feelings of loneliness. Both peer acceptance and friendships affect a child's self-esteem and psychological adjustment; even popular children can experience feelings of loneliness which are mitigated more by intimate friendships more than by popularity with peers.

Children may develop problems because of a lack of good peer relationships and in struggling with peer relationships miss out on opportunities to learn social skills and develop their confidence. School can be an intensely difficult experience in this context. However, the nature of some mental health problems makes it more difficult for children to develop effective peer relationships. In ADHD, for example, children's inability to manage their impulsivity may lead to aggressive responses and subsequent rejection by peers. The inability to manage social relationships is likely to increase their *differentness*, thereby affecting peer relationships (Asher *et al.* 1982). Orsmond *et al.* (2004) found that for young people with autism, greater participation in social and recreational activities was predicted by individual characteristics (such as greater functional independence, less impairment in social skills and higher levels of internalizing behaviours) and by environmental factors (such as greater maternal social activity, greater number of services used and inclusion in integrated settings while in school).

Peer relationships can have negative as well as positive influences on a young person. The need for acceptance, peer approval and wanting to belong may mean that some young people will engage in risky behaviour or behaviour that runs against the expectations for that young person. Smoking is a very good example of negative peer pressure. Young people may have to withstand considerable pressure to resist joining in. Group bullying is another example where young people in a group behave very differently to how they might if they were alone.

Wider cultural and political contexts

As mentioned earlier, one also has to be aware of wider social and political contexts (such as war) that neither clinicians nor families can influence. The factors below may also be less amenable to influence.

Culture

Culture itself does not cause mental health problems. However, understanding cultural contexts may help clinicians present issues in ways that are acceptable to families, thereby making them amenable to intervention. There are very few culturally specific problems but certain disorders are more likely to occur in some contexts than others. For example, the eating dis-order anorexia nervosa is more common in western contexts. Children living within the Western environment (the UK) show different prevalence rates for anorexia, with those of Indian girls being considerably lower than other groups (Office for National Statistics 2004). However, the small numbers of ethnic children represented makes it difficult to be conclusive. Culture may influence the development of mental health problems by its impact on how gender roles, parenting styles and so on are enacted. Culture and religion may also influence how mental health problems and the interventions used to address them are viewed (Yeh *et al.* 2004).

Different cultural practices and belief systems give rise to different challenges in the care of a child. This amazing diversity also means there is a need to be careful in the way we use categories/labels that have been derived from studies on mainly white middle-class European or North American samples. A good example of this point is Chao's (1994) study of parenting styles in Chinese American and European American families. Chao suggested that the word 'authoritarian' had different connotations for the two groups: for most Europeans it implies dominance, control and even hostility, whereas within Chinese systems of socialization an emphasis on parental control and child obedience is accompanied by 'a supportive, highly involved and physically close mother-child relationship' (Chao 1994: 12). Chao found that Chinese American mothers differed from European American mothers on 'training', a pattern of parenting that is important to the Chinese culture.

Younger children will often accept what they are told about their families and family values. As they move into adolescence, wider cultural expectations may influence their devel-oping sense of identity, leading them to question parental/family values. There is often an assumption that differences between parents and young people are more likely in ethnic minority families. The explanation given is that the parents may hold views consistent with their ethnic origin, whereas adolescents face the task of integrating the wider culture in which they have grown up with their family's culture. This is often presented as eastern cultures having a more collective sense of identity, while western cultures are more focused on individuals. In practice, most families have a unique culture of their own. Cultural practices often vary between the private (usually the home) and public domains (school or work). Different families and young people manage in diverse ways. Some may integrate the culture of origin and the culture of the new country, others may switch between cultures depending on the context, and still others may fuse elements of both cultures to produce a unique culture of their own.

Issues that may give rise to problems are:

- pressures to conform to their family's religion or other practices that do not sit comfortably with the young person;
- pressures to conform to expected gender roles (boys wanting to pursue careers generally considered to be in the female domain such as nursing and child care, and vice versa);
- pressures to conform to social norms (e.g. the expectation that a young person will go on to further education despite this not being what they want);
- pressures to conform to family expectations that differ from what the young person wants (e.g. an expectation that the young person will work in the family business);
- sexual orientation;
- impending forced marriages;
- difficulty in reconciling the culture in the private and public domains.

Young people may respond by challenging their parents, rebelling and becoming non-compliant, self-harming and/or becoming moody and withdrawn. They may become depressed especially if they feel there is no possibility of resolution.

Socio-economic disadvantage

Poverty and socio-economic disadvantage are strongly correlated with the development of mental health problems in both children and adults. Sometimes it is assumed that the risk is genetic, whereas the environment may be the key risk factor. Poverty may compromise parenting resources, bringing with it unstable and fragmented communities. In terms of the macrosystem, one of the most pernicious factors that impact on children and families is poverty. UNICEF (2005) looked at 24 of the 30 states in the Organization for Economic Cooperation and Development (OECD) and found that, over the past decade, the number of children living in poverty had risen in 17 countries. Even in the few countries where deprivation is declining the rate can remain high – as is the case in the USA, where about 22 per cent of children under 18 are still living in relative poverty. Similarly, the UK has 15 per cent of the child population below the poverty line despite government campaigns which have led to a 10 per cent drop. The figures refer to relative poverty defined as households with income per head below 50 per cent of the national average.

Poverty affects both parents and children. In parents, poverty may increase stress, affecting parental styles (e.g. they may use autocratic parenting styles) and nurturing behaviour. For children, poverty is associated with higher rates of environmentally induced illnesses, intellectual and physical problems, as well as greater risk for later mental health difficulties, especially depression (Gilman *et al.* 2003).

Summary

In this chapter we have considered the factors that may play a part in the development of child mental health problems. The important point to remember is that rarely, if ever, does a single factor cause mental health problems. Rather, it is the complex interplay of social, psychological and biological factors that leads to the development of difficulties. Understanding the aetiology may help in preventing the development of some problems, managing others and planning effective interventions. Children's behaviour influences the way people respond towards them, thus increasing or decreasing the impact of psycho-social risk. The risk often lies not in the variable per se, but in how it interacts with other factors such as family life. Warm and supportive relationships with at least one parent may limit (or protect against) the impact of disadvantage. The wider community plays a role in maintaining (or undermining) psychological health: strong attachments to adults outside the immediate family improve individual resilience in the face of family adversity; positive school experiences make it more likely that young people will develop a tendency to plan life decisions; the quality of peer relationships influences psycho-social risk.

Now complete the exercise presented in Box 3.6.

| **Box 3.6** **Exercise** | • Consider the child or young person whom you reflected on in Box 3.1.
• What might be the possible risk factors for mental health problems?
• What, if any, are the social, psychological or biological factors?
• Can you differentiate between factors that are causing the problem and those that maintain it?
• Are your thoughts the same on having completed this chapter, or are there factors you had not previously considered? Is the weight you give to factors as cause or consequence the same?
• Discuss your findings with a colleague and see how much agreement there is between you. |

References

Asher, S.R., Renshaw, P.D. and Hymel, S. (1982) Peer relations and the development of social skills, in S.G. Moore and C.R. Cooper (eds) *The Young Child: Reviews Of Research*, Vol. 3. Washington, DC: National Association for the Education of Young Children.

Baumrind, D. (1966) Effects of authoritative parental control on child behavior, *Child Development*, 37(4): 887–907.

Belsky, J. and Vondra, J. (1989) Lessons from child abuse: the development of parenting, in D. Cicchetti and V. Carlson (eds) *Child Maltreatment*. Cambridge: Cambridge University Press.

Bond, L., Carlin, J., Thomas, L., Rubin, K. and Patton, G. (2001) Does bullying cause emotional problems: a prospective study of young teenagers, *British Medical Journal*, 323(7311): 480–4.

Bowlby, J. (1969) *Attachment and Loss, Vol. 1, Attachment*. London: Hogarth Press.

Brodsky, B.S. and Stanley, B. (2008) Adverse childhood experiences and suicidal behaviour, *Psychiatric Clinics of North America*, 31(2): 223–35.

Bronfenbrenner, U. (1979) Contexts of child rearing: problems and prospects, *American Psychologist*, 34: 644–850.

Chao, R. (1994). Beyond parental control and authoritarian parenting style: understanding Chinese parenting through the cultural notion of training, *Child Development*, 65: 1111–19.

Chess, S. and Thomas, A.T. (1999) *Goodness of Fit: Clinical Applications from Infancy through Life*. New York: Routledge.

Cooper, P.J. and Murray, L. (1997) Prediction, detection, and treatment of postnatal depression, *Archives of Disease in Childhood*, 77(2): 97–9.

Das Gupta, P. (1995) Growing up in families, in P. Barnes (ed.) *Personal, Social and Emotional Development*. Oxford: Blackwell.

DfES (Department for Education and Skills) (2003) *Every Child Matters*. London: DfES.

Dunn, J. (1988) Sibling influences on childhood development, *Journal of Child Psychology and Psychiatry*, 29: 119–27.

Dwairy, M. (2004) Parenting styles and mental health of Palestinian-Arab adolescents in Israel, *Transcultural Psychiatry*, 41(2): 233–52.

Dwairy, M. and Menshar, K.E. (2006) Parenting style, individuation and mental health of Egyptian adolescents, *Journal of Adolescence*, 29: 103–17.

Eiduson, B.T., Kornfein M., Zimmerman, I.L. and Weisner, T.S. (1999) Comparative socialization practices in traditional and alternative families, in M. Lamb (ed.) *Non-Traditional Families: Parenting and Child Development*. Hillsdale, NJ: Erlbaum.

Elias, M,J., Zins, J.E., Weissberg, R.P., Frey, K.S., Greenberg, M.T., Haynes, N.M., Kessler, R., Schwab-Stone, M.E. and Shriver, T.P. (1997) *Promoting Social and Emotional Learning: Guidelines for Educator*. Alexandria, VA: Association for Supervision and Curriculum Development.

Gilman, S.E., Kawachi, I., Fitzmaurice, G.M. and Buka, S.L. (2003) Family disruption in childhood and risk of adult depression, *American Journal of Psychiatry*, 16: 939–46.

Gordon, J. and Grant, G. (1997) *How We Feel: An Insight into the Emotional World of Teenagers*. London: Jessica Kingsley.

Green, H., McGinnity, A., Meltzer, H., Ford, T. and Goodman, R. (2005) *Mental Health of Children and Adolescents in Great Britain*. London: Palgrave Macmillan.

Johnson, D.W. and Johnson, R.T. (2004) The three Cs of promoting social and emotional learning, in J.E. Zins, R.P. Weissberg, M.C. Wang and H.J. Walberg (eds) *Building Academic Success on Social and Emotional Learning: What Does the Research Say?* New York: Teachers College Press.

Koenen, K.C., Moffitt, T.E., Roberts, A.L., Martin, L.T., Kubzansky, L., Harrington, H., Poulton, R. and Caspi, A. (2009) Childhood IQ and adult mental disorders: a test of the cognitive reserve hypothesis, *The American Journal of Psychiatry*, 166: 50–7.

Lonigan, C.J., Phillips, B.M. and Hooe, E.S. (2003) Relations of positive and negative affectivity to anxiety and depression in children: evidence from a latent variable longitudinal study, *Journal of Consulting and Clinical Psychology*, 71(3): 465–81.

Macoby, E.E. and Martin, J.A. (1983) Socialisation in the context of the family: parent-child interaction, in P.H. Mussen and E.M. Hetherington (eds) *Handbook of Child Psychology, Volume 4, Socialisation, Personality and Social Development*, 4th edn. New York: Wiley.

Manassis, K. (2001) Child-parent relations: attachment and anxiety disorders, in W.K. Silverman and P.D.A. Treffers (eds) *Anxiety Disorders in Children and Adolescents: Research, Assessment and Intervention*. Cambridge: Cambridge University Press.

Manning, C. and Gregoire, A. (2006) Effects of parental mental illness on children, *Psychiatry*, 5(1): 10–12.

Mortimore, P. (1995) The positive effects of schooling, in M. Rutter (ed.) *Psychosocial Disturbances in Young People: Challenges for Prevention*. Cambridge: Cambridge University Press.

Office for National Statistics (2004) *Mental Health of Children and Young People, Great Britain*, www.statistics.gov.uk/downloads/theme_health/GB2004.pdf, accessed 2 July 2009.

Orsmond, G.I., Krauss, M.W. and Seltzer, M.M. (2004) Peer relationships and social and recreational activities among adolescent and adults with autism, *Journal of Autism and Developmental Disorders*, 34(3): 245–56.

Pawluck, D.E. and Gorey, K.M. (1998) Secular trends in the incidence of anorexia nervosa: integrative review of population based studies, *International Journal of Eating Disorders*, 23: 347–52.

Pickens, J. and Field, T. (1993) Facial expressivity in infants of depressed mothers, *Developmental Psychology*, 29(6): 986–88.

Prior, V. and Glaser, D. (2006) *Understanding Attachment and Attachment Disorders: Theory, Evidence and Practice*. London: Jessica Kingsley.

Sanders, R. (2004) *Sibling Relationships: Theory and Issues for Practice*. Basingstoke: Palgrave Macmillan.

Schaffer, H.R. (1996) *Social Development*. Oxford: Blackwell.

Schaffer, H.R. (1998) *Making Decisions About Children*. Oxford: Blackwell.

Surgeon General's Office (2009) *Mental Health: A Report of the Surgeon General*, www.surgeongeneral.gov/library/mentalhealth/chapter3/sec2.html, accessed 20 January 2009.

UNICEF (2005) *Innocenti Report: Child Poverty in Rich Countries*, http://www.unicef.org.uk/press/pdf/Report Card6.pdf, accessed 20 January 2009.

Yeh, M., Hough, R., McCabe, K., Lau, A. and Garland, A. (2004) Parental beliefs about the causes of child problems: exploring racial/ethnic patterns, *Journal of the American Academy of Child and Adolescent Psychiatry*, 43(5): 605–12.

Zins, J.E., Bloodworth. M.R., Weissberg, R.P. and Walberg, H.J. (2004) The scientific base linking social and emotional learning in school success, in J.E. Zins, R.P. Weissberg, M.C. Wang and H.J. Walberg (eds) *Building Academic Success on Social and Emotional Learning: What Does the Research Say?* New York: Teachers College Press.

Further reading

Phoenix, A. and Husain, A.F. (2007) *Parenting: Ethnicity, a Review*. York: Joseph Rowntree Foundation.

Vostanis, P. (ed.) *Mental Health Interventions and Services for Vulnerable Children and Young People*. London: Jessica Kingsley.

4 Legal and ethical considerations in CAMH

Sharon Leighton

Key features
- Explores some of the legal and ethical considerations associated with clinical decision-making in order to demonstrate that child and adolescent mental health (CAMH) nursing is both an art and a science.
- Demonstrates how reflecting on the issues of consent, capacity, competence and confidentiality influences making treatment decisions with children.

Introduction

It is important to clarify at the beginning that I am writing from the perspective of a clinician, being neither a lawyer nor an ethicist. This chapter provides a practical example of how the art and science of CAMH nursing can come together in practice.

The aim is to reflect on some of the ethical challenges faced by practitioners by exploring some of the contradictions in law associated with child care. The statutory requirements identified in various Acts can sometimes appear contradictory, giving practitioners a minefield to navigate. It might be helpful to bear in mind that because something is legal does not make it ethical and vice versa.

Aristotle viewed *considered reflection* as the heart of ethics on the grounds that a reflective process should be undertaken every time there are conclusions to be reached about the worth of human activity (Kaufmann 1998). Seedhouse (2005: 136) identifies that:

> ethical analysis is a matter of reflecting on evidence and values, with the genuine intent of finding the most reasonable solution to our problems . . . [but] there are no answers that are truly ethical and no clear ultimate solutions.

Moreover, considered reflection involves generating questions, living with uncertainty and discomfort, and coping with failures and mistakes (Stott *et al.* 2006); in other words, living life.

Western health care is now increasingly underpinned by policies, procedures and protocols. However, individual practitioners need to be able to reflect on the ethical and legal aspects of their decision-making. While professional codes of conduct, evidence-based practice, individual values, the definition of concepts and changes in health and social care are essential considerations when making decisions, they are not the focus of this discussion. However, consideration of individual values will be evident when undertaking the chapter exercises.

Furthermore, it is worth noting that the professional code of practice requires a nurse to work within their level of competence, but does not explicitly establish what that involves (NMC 2008). Such ethical codes of conduct with their universal and abstract competencies underpin professional autonomy within the modern National Health Service (NHS) and allow professionals to be regulated at a distance while holding them individually accountable (Kennedy and Kennedy 2004). Given that the actions of individual nurses will be strongly influenced by managerial and political factors, the feasibility of individual accountability is questionable.

The legal framework

The legal framework in the UK consists of common law and statute law. Common law is based on custom and the corresponding legal system developed through decisions of courts and similar tribunals rather than through legislative statutes. In health care it defines the rights and responsibilities of patients and health care practitioners in areas not covered by legislation. The guiding principles are that there is a degree of urgency plus safety/protection issues, that the intervention must end when the emergency situation is resolved, and the rights of the patient must be protected at all times (Martin 2006).

Box 4.1 Read the following case scenario and then consider the questions posed.
Exercise

Sam, 14 years, is brought to accident & emergency (A&E) by his girlfriend, having cut his wrists. He does not want to be treated, insisting that he wants to leave A&E and go home.

- Can Sam be held in A&E and treated by doctors against his will?
- Can he be treated given that his parents are not present?

Statute law (i.e. laws passed by Parliament) in relation to children includes the key legislation highlighted in Box 4.2. I do not propose to go through the legislation, other than to refer to pertinent issues and to relate theory to practice.

Box 4.2 Key legislation relating to children

- Children Act 1989, implemented 1991.
- UN Convention on Rights of the Child 1989 (ratified by UK government 1999).
- Sex Offenders Act 1997.
- Crime and Disorder Act 1998.
- Human Rights Act 1998, implemented October 2000.
- Children (Leaving Care) Act 2000.
- Children Act 2004.
- Mental Health Act 1983, as amended by the Mental Health Act 2007, implemented 2008.

Children Act

The focus of the Children Act 1989 is the welfare of the child. Its philosophical underpinnings include: the child's welfare is paramount; children are generally better looked after in their natural family; courts should intervene only if it is clearly in a child's best interests. Under the Children Act a child in need is identified as unlikely to achieve, maintain, or have the opportunity of achieving/maintaining reasonable standards of health/development without appropriate provision of services by the local authority; their health or development are likely to be significantly/further impaired without such services; or they are disabled (Children Act 1989, Part III, Section 17(10)).

The most recent Children Act goes beyond child protection issues and considers the context in which children live. Under the Children Act 2004, four main aims for action are identified: supporting parents/carers; early intervention and effective protection; accountability and integration (local, regional, national); workforce reform. A duty is placed on key statutory agencies to safeguard and promote the welfare of children, ensuring that others providing services on their behalf follow the same approach and provision is made for pooled funding of children's services. The underlying justification is to prevent some children from becoming children in need through the joint planning of non-stigmatizing services by the statutory agencies, community organizations (e.g. schools and CAMHS), the voluntary sector and children and their families.

Box 4.3 **Exercise**	• Reflect on what might be the positive and negative outcomes of commissioning specialist CAMHS for vulnerable children along with all other services such as education, and/or social services, for this group.

Human Rights Act

The Human Rights Act 1998 established a statutory framework for applying rights contained in the European Convention on Human Rights, to domestic law. Article 8 is discussed as an exemplar: *the right to respect for private and family life* is a qualified right whereby interference in family life is allowed if it is lawful, serves a legitimate purpose, is necessary in democratic society and is not discriminatory (e.g. for the prevention of disorder or crime, protection of health or protection of rights/freedom of others).

Box 4.4 Case scenario

Josh, 15 years, lives with his mum and sister (Sarah, 12). His dad is serving a prison sentence for the attempted murder of Josh's mum. During his time in prison he has sent many letters threatening to kill the family when he gets out. Release is imminent and Josh feels increasingly frustrated by a perceived lack of concern from agencies involved with the family. At a school drop-in clinic he tells the school nurse of his plans to take the law into his own hands.

• Can the school nurse contravene Article 8?
• If so, what are the justifications?

Making treatment decisions with children

This is an area fraught with legal and ethical considerations. Here, the reader is offered an opportunity to reflect on some of the pertinent issues by relating theory to practice. The issues associated with treatment decisions which are highlighted include consent, capacity, competence and confidentiality.

In law, a child is defined as 'a person under the age of 18' (Children Act 1989). However, the Mental Capacity Act (2005) defines adults as aged 16 years and above.

Consent

Consent is the act of saying one is willing to do something or agreeing that somebody else can do something (e.g. agreeing to treatment). It does not always have to be in writing. However, to be valid it requires the following: capacity to be able to make a decision; sufficient information to make a decision, made of the individual's own free will, free from pressure from others.

Informed consent is a complex and controversial concept when applied to children and consent to medical treatment (Bartholomew 1996; Goodwin *et al.* 2000; Paul 2004). The law recognizes that, as children develop, they acquire the capacity to make personal decisions for themselves, including decisions on medical treatment. The Gillick case and S.8(1) of the Family Law Reform Act (1969) are evidence of this.

Under the Children Act 1989, parental responsibility (PR) refers to all rights, duties, powers, responsibilities and authorities which by law the parent of a child has in relation to that child and their property. It covers decisions made regarding medical treatment. A child aged 16 years or over can consent to any medical treatment, while one who is under 16 years requires the consent of those with PR (except in a medical emergency). Competence to consent to treatment is not defined in the Children Act 1989, and yet *Gillick competence* is used as a measure of a child's ability to consent. This provides an example of how statute and common law can contradict each other.

Gillick provides ambiguous guidelines as to what constitutes capacity to consent, and does not address the issue of mentally disturbed or disordered children (Bridge 1997). Furthermore, a Gillick-competent child may give consent to assessment/treatment but can have a refusal over-ruled by parents or those *in loco parentis* on the grounds of lack of competence. However, under the Mental Health Act 2007, 16- or 17-year-olds can refuse to be admitted informally to hospital for mental health treatment, even if their parents are willing to consent. Box 4.6 highlights the issues associated with children and consent.

Box 4.5 **Exercise**	• Consider what might impact on a child's capability to consent to psychiatric treatment.

Box 4.6 Children and consent to treatment

- Gillick competence provides unclear guidelines regarding what constitutes 'capacity to consent'.
- Gillick competence does not address the issue of mental disturbance/illness. A child must be able to understand the nature of proposed treatment, possible side-effects and the consequences of not receiving the treatment.
- It is possible for a child to be found competent to make a decision regarding treatment that might have minor consequences, but not to make a decision where major consequences are involved.
- A child's right to consent cannot be overruled by anyone with PR, but a court can override it.
- A child may give consent to assessment/treatment, but can have a refusal over-ruled by those with PR on the grounds of lack of competence.
- As long as a person with PR consents to treatment on a child's behalf, the child has no right to refuse, even if judged competent.

- In practice, courts always find incompetence when a child refuses life-saving treatment.
- 16- or 17-year-olds can refuse to be admitted informally to hospital for mental health treatment, even if their parents are willing to consent.

Capacity

Capacity is the legal term which represents a patient's ability to consent. It consists of the following abilities: understanding and retaining information about a proposed treatment and the consequences of not having it; weighing up information; making a free choice. This provides a limited picture, as the focus is solely on the decision-making ability shown in this situation. Under the Mental Capacity Act 2005, all adults (i.e. people aged 16 years and older) are assumed to have the capacity to make their own decisions, unless there is evidence to the contrary. However, at present there is no accurate way to determine when an individual has achieved 'autonomous capacity'. Reder and Fitzpatrick (1998: 103) point out that:

Children's sufficient understanding is deemed a critical factor in determining their capacity to consent to treatment . . . However, the concept has remained undefined . . . it should refer not only to the child's cognitive development, but also to the influence of personal and interpersonal conflicts.

Furthermore, acknowledgement needs to be given to the possible effects of traumatic experiences on a child's feelings and values, as well as on their developing brain (Dickenson and Jones 1996; Le Doux 2002). Such effects can impinge on a child's ability to make a decision regarding consent to treatment.

Aiken (2001) suggests that in the interests of consistency and fairness, decision-making should include all relevant individuals (i.e. parents/carer, child) who have attained the cognitive and volitional capacity to deliberate and act on a set of values.

Competence

Competence is a clinical not a legal term. A clinical concept is useful as it enables clinicians to consider several factors, which are not legally recognized, in assessing ability to consent: ability to make reasonably consistent decisions over time; decisions consistent with previously expressed opinions; personality factors; decision-making with regard to current and future circumstances and risks; the effects of emotional states and illness on decision-making ability. However, there is no standard or agreed definition of the clinical concept of competence. Beauchamp and Childress (1989) define competence as the ability to perform specific tasks. Tan and Jones (2001) define it as the ability of a person to consent to treatment. Leighton (2007: 51), on the other hand, puts it this way:

A simple working definition is that a person is competent if they are able to achieve what they set out to achieve – for example, if a child can demonstrate that they understand what is being proposed in terms of therapy, potential consequences of receiving/not receiving treatment, then they are competent to make a decision. However, their competence could be improved by providing alternative options to the treatment proposed.

The concept of competency in relation to a child's consent to psychiatric treatment can be viewed as a multi-faceted and complex interaction involving: the developmental stage of the child and its effect on cognitive ability and rationality; their social environment and previous experience; their relationship with the professional, as well as with their family; information presented to them about the treatment, as well as their understanding of that information; and their mental state at the time of making the decision (Batten 1996; Reder and Fitzpatrick 1998; Paul 2004).

Capacity and development

The law recognizes that as children develop, they acquire the capacity to make their own personal decisions, including for medical treatment. However, the legally imposed age boundaries used to distinguish the 'evolving capacities' of the child, and to represent the transition from child to adult status, are not necessarily synonymous with the actual level of maturity and competence. Differences in competence are relative rather than absolute; most adults are only competent in a few aspects of life. Furthermore, competence is context-specific. Nevertheless, a child's identity will be less established than an adult's and their decisions based on less secure wishes, intentions, motives, emotions and values (Dickenson and Jones 1996).

Adults who are deemed competent to consent to treatment are not considered incompetent if they refuse treatment. Moreover, adults are presumed competent to refuse or consent to medical treatment regardless of mental illness; but whether or not they are mentally ill, children are believed incompetent should they decide to refuse treatment. They can however be considered competent if they give consent to treatment where their carers decline the option. Providing that someone with parental responsibility for a child consents to treatment on their behalf, the child has no right to refuse consent, whether or not judged competent (e.g. social services on behalf of a looked-after child). Despite rulings that capacity and not age is the relevant factor in determining competence, practice indicates that children are presumed incompetent and must prove otherwise, while the opposite is true for those over 18 (Reder and Fitzpatrick 1998; Paul 2004).

Box 4.7 Case scenario: the difference between consent and competency

Ellie is 15 years old and presents with a moderate depressive illness. The management plan suggested includes the use of an antidepressant. Ellie states that she would prefer not to use medication. Her parents urge you to persuade her that this is necessary and that she must do as they request as she is under 16. You have to explain to Ellie's parents that Ellie has the competency to decline consent for the use of antidepressants and her wishes have to be taken into consideration. Just because Ellie does not agree with the management plan, her views cannot be discounted.

Box 4.8 Considerations if a child refuses treatment deemed to be in their best interests

- Age and developmental level of understanding.
- Capacity.
- Opinion of child.
- Who has PR?
- Opinion of person/agency with PR.
- Legal framework.

The Mental Health Act 2007 brings into effect a number of amendments to the Mental Health Act 1983 and the Mental Capacity Act 2005. In relation to CAMHS the issues include: 16- or 17-year-olds can refuse to be admitted informally to hospital for mental health treatment, even if their parents are willing to consent; children (if admitted) to be admitted to age-appropriate settings, assessed by a medical practitioner with specialist training in CAMH (except in an emergency) and the *responsible clinician* to be a child specialist (except in an emergency). The rationale for this is that these young people do not end up in effect detained in hospital against their will, without the protections given to people who are formally detained under the Mental Health Act.

Box 4.9 **Exercise**	• Given that detentions under the Mental Health Act are normally seen as an emergency admission, how might that affect the requirement that adolescents be admitted to age-appropriate settings, and be looked after by CAMH professionals? • Define an 'age-appropriate setting'.

Confidentiality

There is no definition in statute law in England or Wales regarding confidential relationships (Hamilton 2005). The central tenet of the Children Act 1989 is that of *significant harm*. Bentovim (1991: 29) defines 'significant harm' as: 'a compilation of significant events . . . acute and long-standing, which interact with . . . ongoing development and interrupt, alter or impair physical and psychological development'.

Social services are under a statutory obligation to act when there is reasonable cause to suspect that a child is suffering, or is likely to suffer, significant harm according to the Children Act 1989. All agencies working with children are obliged to work in partnership to promote their welfare and to protect them from abuse and neglect. The safety and welfare of the child is paramount and necessitates sharing information about suspected abuse with statutory agencies (DoH 1999). Therefore, although some relationships are automatically seen as confidential (e.g. doctor/patient; counsellor/client), the need to protect children from significant harm means that no service for them can guarantee absolute confidentiality (Hamilton 2005). Given that establishing a good working relationship with a child often requires assurance of confidentiality, boundaries need to be made clear before a child (and their family) begins to make use of a service.

When deciding whether or not to disclose confidential information, a question arises as to whether the proposed disclosure is a proportionate response to the need to protect the welfare of the child. Where disclosure is deemed necessary, the amount of confidential information disclosed, and the number of people to whom it is divulged, should be no more than is strictly necessary to meet the public interest in protecting the health and well-being of the child.

Box 4.10 **Exercise**	• What impact does the Human Rights Act 1998 have on confidentiality? Would disclosure be justified under Article 8.2? • What if the child disclosed sexual abuse that occurred several years ago and there is no contact with abuser?

The final task is for the reader to complete the following exercise. This may be done individually or in discussion with colleagues.

Box 4.11 Case scenarios involving legal and ethical issues

Read the following case scenarios and then consider these questions which illustrate the complexity of the issues involved and the fact that there are no easy answers.

- What do you decide to do?
- How do you justify your decision legally?
- How do you justify your decision ethically?
- How might this decision affect your relationship with the child?
- How might this decision affect your relationship with their parents/carers?

Case scenario 1

Becky, aged 15, has lived with her paternal grandparents on an informal basis since infancy. Her father has long-term mental health problems and relies heavily on the paternal grandmother for support. The mother left the family 14 years ago. Becky was referred to CAMHS with symptoms of anxiety and depression.

Both Becky and her grandmother request that copies of correspondence are sent to the grandmother and not to the father.

Case scenario 2

You work in a community CAMHS team. James, aged 16, was admitted to an inpatient unit with depression. As part of his planned discharge you agree to re-establish contact and undertake three sessions with him before the next review meeting. It becomes increasingly obvious over the sessions that James is not coping as well as he is leading others to believe. You have to decide whether to inform the parents at this stage and risk James not disclosing any further information, or to share the information at the review meeting.

Summary

Exploration of some of the legal and ethical issues associated with clinical decision-making demonstrates that CAMH nursing is both an art and a science. The art is evident in how ethical analysis is used as a vehicle for reflecting on the legalities of consent, capacity, competence and confidentiality (the evidence), in order to make treatment decisions with children experiencing mental health problems (the science).

References

Aiken, W. (2001) Moral reflection on adolescent decision making? *Community Ethics, Special Supplement* 7(1), http://www.pitt.edu/~cep/documents/Vol7No1.pdf, accessed 1 August 2006.

Bartholomew, T. (1996) Challenging assumptions about young people's competence: clearing the pathway to policy? Paper presented at the fifth Australian Family Research conference, www.aifs.gov.au, accessed 1 August 2006.

Batten, D. (1996) Informed consent by children and adolescents to psychiatric treatment, *Australian and New Zealand Journal of Psychiatry*, 30: 623–32.

Beauchamp, T. and Childress, J. (1989) *Principles of Biomedical Ethics*, 3rd edn. Oxford: Oxford University Press.

Bentovim, A. (1991) Significant harm in context, in M. Adcock, R. White and A. Hollows (eds) *Significant Harm*. Croydon: Significant Publications.

Bridge, C. (1997) Adolescents and mental disorder: who consents to treatment? *Medical Law International*, 3: 51–74.

Dickenson, D. and Jones, D. (1996) True wishes: the philosophy and developmental psychology of children's informed consent, *Philosophy, Psychiatry and Psychology*, 2: 287–303.

DoH (Department of Health) (1999) *Working Together to Safeguard Children: A Guide to Inter-agency Working to Safeguard and Promote the Welfare of Children*. London: DoH.

Goodwin, M., Bickerton, A., Parsons, R. and Lask, B. (2000) Paediatric heart/heart-lung transplantation: a systemic perspective on assessment and preparation, *International Journal of Psychiatry in Clinical Practice*, 4: 93–9.

Hamilton, C. (2005) *Working with Young People: Legal Responsibility and Liability*, 6th edn. Colchester: The Children's Legal Centre.

Kaufmann, W. (1998) *Aristotle: Nicomachean Ethics*. New York: Dover Thrift Editions.

Kennedy, C. and Kennedy, P. (2004) The moral management of nursing labour power: conceptualising control and resistance, in S. Fleetwood and S. Ackroyd (eds) *Critical Realist Applications in Organisation and Management Studies*. London: Routledge.

Le Doux, J. (2002) *Synaptic Self: How our Brains Become Who We Are*. New York: Penguin.

Leighton, S. (2007) Ethical issues in working therapeutically with vulnerable children, in P. Vostanis (ed.) *Mental Health Interventions and Services for Vulnerable Children and Young People*. London: Jessica Kingsley.

Martin, E.A. (2006) *A Dictionary of Law*. Oxford: Oxford University Press.

NMC (Nursing and Midwifery Council) (2008) *The Code: Standards of Conduct, Performance and Ethics for Nurses and Midwives*, www.nmc-uk.org/aArticle.aspx?ArticleID=3057, accessed 20 August 2008.

Paul, M. (2004) Decision-making about children's mental health care: ethical challenges, *Advances in Psychiatric Treatment*, 10: 301–11.

Reder, P. and Fitzpatrick, G. (1998) What is sufficient understanding? *Clinical Child Psychology and Psychiatry*, 3: 103–13.

Seedhouse, D. (2005) *Values-Based Decision-Making for the Caring Professionals*. Chichester: Wiley.

Stott, L., Nissin, R., Dent, H. and Golding, K.S. (2006) Travelling hopefully – the journey continues, in K.S. Golding, H. Dent, R. Nissim and L. Stott (eds) *Thinking Psychologically About Children who are Looked After and Adopted*. Chichester: Wiley.

Tan, J. and Jones, D. (2001) Children's consent, *Current Opinion in Psychiatry*, 14: 303–7.

5 Nursing assessment in CAMHS

Nisha Dogra and Laurence Baldwin

> **Key features**
> - Outline of the principles of nursing assessments in CAMHS.
> - The key components of a nursing assessment.
> - How to ensure cultural issues are appropriately addressed.
> - Focus on risk assessment and safeguarding.
> - Presentation of Calgary family assessment and intervention models.

Introduction

In this chapter we begin by exploring the role of the nurse within child and adolescent mental health services (CAMHS) in the assessment of child mental health problems. We then describe what constitutes a CAMHS nursing assessment and highlight key components that warrant particular attention as they may be less familiar. There is a focus on developmental assessments and tools that may help nurses undertake development histories that enable them to best help the child. We consider how every assessment can be tailored for each family and principles that can be applied to ensure that the cultural needs of every child and family are assessed. We outline the contents and process for some specialist assessments such as risk assessments, as these are sometimes specifically requested. Family assessments are not covered in this chapter as they are dealt with in Chapter 7. However, we do discuss models that help integrate systems theory with CAMHS nursing.

Key principles of nursing assessments

Much of the material covered in this chapter may also be used by other professions, but we suggest that nurses need to consider what they contribute, by virtue of their nursing training, to the assessment of children, young people and their families. In some cases this may be quite clear – that you are acting, for example, in a specific role, or with a specific aim in mind. You may be part of a family therapy clinic, and the nature of your assessment will then naturally reflect the systemic way in which you are working. At other times, however, it may be that there is less of a directive framework or specific guidance for the work you are doing with a child, young person or family. While it is important for nurses that they remain flexible and are able to work in a variety of ways, it is also important to be clear about what you are doing, and with what aim at any given time. In the past some nurses have described their work as 'eclectic', by which they ought to mean they are drawing on a range of different approaches to therapeutic work. If this is so in your case, you should be clear which element is being used at any given time, rather than using it as an excuse for muddling along with-out a clear model in your head. Nursing models, for example, may come with a variety of different theoretical orientations underpinning their practice, and we will look briefly at some of these.

Evans (1999) points out that nursing roles may be multi-faceted and dependent on the task being performed at any given time. She notes six discrete areas which nurses will recognize from mental health nursing traditions as being potential aspects of nursing strength within a wider assessment framework:

- *creator of a therapeutic environment* – more obvious in residential settings, but nurses may also need to stress the need for the creation of a therapeutic environment at home or in other settings;
- *socializing agent* – modelling or teaching social skills within defined socially acceptable limits;
- *counsellor, parent surrogate and teacher* – varied applications within residential and community settings according to the role required;
- *technician* – in particular with regard to medication administration and psycho-education about medication management;
- *case manager* – increasingly nurses have total management responsibility for cases within services – this may include roles as case coordinator under the care programme approach, or as lead professional for the Common Assessment Framework (in England);
- *advocate* – either in individual cases or as part of a wider role within and across organizations or in multi-agency forums.

This fits in with the wider task of applying skills learnt within other areas of nursing practice (in the UK either as a mental health or paediatric trained nurse) to a specifically CAMH setting. Johnson and Baggett (1995: 15), for example, note that nursing skill in assessing child and adolescent problems is 'based on cognitive and affective abilities that allow the nurse to make high-level inferences about psychiatric and psychosocial problems'. It is also clear that nurses are one of the groups that have the most direct contact with children and young people with mental health problems (McDougall 2006: 11), and they should be in a position to use their nursing skills to offer quality patient-centred care. Although there is no overall consensus as to what exactly is the underlying conceptual framework of mental health nursing, there is strong evidence that most mental health nurses rely on a concept of interpersonal relations, a 'therapeutic relationship' which is developed between the nurse and 'patient'. Barker (1999) locates this within a tradition of nursing initiated by Peplau (1982), and popularized in the UK by Altschul (1972). The role of the nurse in CAMHS, therefore, would be to adapt and use the skills of interpersonal engagement and the therapeutic use of self in a constructive manner within assessment and treatment processes. It is possible that this emphasis, within nursing, on therapeutic engagement and relationships, provides a method of enhancing effective communication and promoting well-being. For example, Brown *et al.* (2006: 185) specifically mention nurses' use of humour as a method of communicating.

We will look at just one model of utilizing nursing skills within a CAMHS context with reference to family assessment later on in the chapter (the Calgary model).

Box 5.1 summarizes the key components of a nursing mental health assessment.

Box 5.1 Key components of a comprehensive nursing CAMHS assessment

- Presenting concerns and history of these.
- Family history.

- Social history.
- Developmental history.
- Integrating cultural issues.
- Mental state examination of child.
- Observation of young people with their carers.
- Risk assessment.
- Formulation and agreeing a care plan.

The assessment framework

It is useful to have an assessment framework, although the details may vary from service to service. There is little evidence or research regarding assessment processes in CAMH nursing (or even in other professional groups), although they have good face validity. We will deal with some of these (developmental history, cultural aspects and risk assessments) in some detail, while briefly highlighting other areas which are well described elsewhere in the nursing literature.

Presenting concerns

It is important to begin by clarifying what the child and/or their carers are expecting and what they know of the service. It is also important to establish their expectations and hopes for the meeting. Consent and confidentiality issues are best addressed early on. It can be helpful for the child to know that there are clear boundaries and that their perspective is as important as those of any adults. It is important also to find out what the child or young person and their family think are the main worries. These may be different from what the referrer has told you, and the relative importance given to different things may vary between different members of the family as well. An accurate history of how long the symptoms or worries have been present may also give a clue to precipitating factors and the need to examine how these have affected people differently.

Family history

Establishing the family history involves identifying who is in the family and what constitutes the family from the child's perspective. As outlined in Chapter 2, fairly broad definitions of family apply within the work of CAMHS. A *genogram* can be a useful way to demonstrate family relationships. Depending on the presenting concerns and history, there may be a need to explore in greater detail how parents themselves were parented. How someone is parented influences how they themselves in turn parent their own children.

Social history

This usually means asking young people about their peer relationships and their interests. As children get older they begin to have more contacts outside of the family. This is a good opportunity to find out what is of interest to the child and can be a good place to begin interviews as it helps engage with the child. The older the child the more important it is to ask about peer activities. Young people may be reluctant to share all aspects of this part of the history with their carers. Drug and alcohol history is an important part of the social history, though again sensitivity may be required in getting honest answers from young people about their use of substances and alcohol.

Developmental assessment

Given that children and young people are developing towards maturation for adulthood, it should come as no surprise that a developmental assessment is a key component of a comprehensive CAMH assessment. A developmental assessment is a structured evaluation of the child's development and a comprehensive assessment needs to cover the key domains – physical, social, emotional, moral and intellectual. Such an assessment is likely to involve several members of the multi-disciplinary team (e.g. formal intellectual assessment is best undertaken by a psychologist who has specific training in this; an assessment of motor development, a component of physical development, may best be undertaken by an occupational therapist). It will also usually involve seeing the child in different contexts and environments.

Some might question which parts of the assessment are the responsibility of CAMHS and which belong to other specialities. However, the reality is that many referrals to CAMHS have developmental components as potential aetiological factors, and even if a developmental assessment has already been undertaken it may be insufficient.

Why is development important to consider?

Consider the symptom of 'inattention and poor concentration'. In a 3-year-old this is not unusual, so a diagnosis of attention deficit hyperactivity disorder (ADHD) is unlikely to be appropriate. However, a child who is 7 years of age and has global developmental delay may still have features of inattention and poor concentration. Only a detailed assessment can clarify the situation and establish whether the child's development is appropriate or not. CAMHS nurses are unlikely to be involved in the investigation of delayed development but may often be the ones who recognize that a child's development is not as it should be. Unless there is a clear understanding of a child's level of functioning and comprehension, not only is it difficult to make an assessment of their presentation, it is also difficult to intervene in the right way.

It is important to highlight children's strengths but it is also only fair to identify their difficulties so that appropriate interventions can be effectively made. Given that individuals with developmental disorders are at risk of behavioural and emotional disturbances as well as psychiatric disorders (Bolton 2001), CAMHS nurses have a responsibility to be aware of the potential of such underlying factors. Although aetiological factors do not always emerge for children with mild global delay or those with specific learning difficulties, the former should be investigated according to evidence-based guidelines (McDonald et al. 2006).

Tools for developmental assessment

Bolton (2001) details the various tools that are available – many of which require specific training and so cannot be used in a clinical assessment. It is useful to have questions for key milestones and if these cause concern a more detailed and perhaps specialist assessment may be warranted.

Box 5.2 Useful screening questions

- Motor: when did the child sit? When did they walk?
- Speech and language: when did the child vocalize? Say words? Their first sentence? There also needs to be a distinction between what a child can understand (comprehension) and what they say (expression).
- Social: how does the child play? Does he or she engage with others?

An indicator that is also clinically invaluable is the Goodenough drawing (Goodenough 1926; Pillitteri 2006) which can be used to assess intelligence, although in CAMHS this use is less likely. A child is essentially asked to draw a person and given points for each characteristic that is present (e.g. head, legs, arms and so on). For every four points one year is added to a base mental age of 3 years. A 5-year-old child should therefore be able to draw a body which has at least eight features (e.g. head, legs, arms, trunk, with shoulders, arms and legs attached to trunk, then attached to the correct part of the trunk, then neck, eyes, nose and mouth, progressively as the child's development advances). This is again not diagnostic but may be an indication that further assessment may be warranted. To date no cultural differences have been found in younger children when the Goodenough Harris 'draw a person test' is used (Dugdale and Chen 1979).

It is important to remember that context is crucial. To develop appropriately a child needs to have both the ability and opportunity to do so. Some children who have experienced neglect may appear developmentally delayed but transfer into a nurturing environment then reveals that they have had no opportunity to develop. Once in the improved environment a child should begin to develop naturally and not require professional intervention.

Although the development assessment of early milestones in adolescents may be less detailed, it can still be relevant. It is not unusual to be referred teenagers who have always had problems in school which have gradually worsened, only to find that they have learning disabilities which have not been identified. The focus of all work to date may have been managing the behaviour rather than trying to establish its cause. Avoiding the label of 'learning disability' is often done at the expense of the child in the long run.

The Vineland's Adaptive Behaviour scales (Sparrow *et al.* 2007) may be a useful tool for CAMHS nurses, especially those working with learning disability teams, to become familiar with.

We will now consider how cultural issues can be integrated into every assessment to ensure that the cultural needs of all families are identified and met.

Integrating cultural issues

There can be an assumption that cultural issues only need to be considered in minority and non-white families. Taking this approach clearly limits the quality of care that patients receive.

Using culture in its broadest sense, as defined for example by the Association of American Medical Colleges (AAMC 1999: 25), may help us deliver tailored care to all families. The definition used is:

Culture is defined by each person in relationship to the group or groups with whom he or she identifies. An individual's cultural identity may be based on heritage as well as individual circumstances and personal choice. Cultural identity may be affected by such factors as race, ethnicity, age, language, country of origin, acculturation, sexual orientation, gender, socioeconomic status, religious/spiritual beliefs, physical abilities, occupation, among others. These factors may impact behaviours such as communication styles, diet preferences, health beliefs, family roles, lifestyle, rituals and decision-making processes. All of these beliefs and practices, in turn can influence how patients and heath care professionals perceive health and illness and how they interact with one another.

Dogra and Karim (2005) argue that this definition is patient-centred and enables patients to decide which of these factors that make up culture are relevant to them. It is probably more effective to have a principle-based approach (Dogra 2003) to ensure that cultural issues are taken on board for all families. There are several reasons for this:

- prevents facts relevant to one individual being assumed to be relevant to others who may appear to be from a similar background;

- should prevent stereotyping of any groups;
- enables the provider to provide quality care irrespective of which factor diversity may be related to;
- works with the central philosophy that young people and their families all bring perspectives which need to be taken into account.

It should be emphasized that currently there is no strong evidence that one type of approach is more effective than another. However, we do know that much of what has been done to date has not been effective (Anderson *et al.* 2003) or has been insufficiently evaluated (Bennett *et al.* 2007).

When working with families in a way which respects their cultural perspectives but also allows you to work within your professional expectations, the following approaches may be helpful.

- Reflect on your own biases and prejudices to ensure that these do not consciously or subconsciously justify less than quality or equal care for all patients.
- As many factors influence a family's understanding of mental health and mental health services, at the outset of any assessment check the family's understanding of what they think is going to happen.
- Be aware that the family may play out expected roles and it may take a lot of encouragement to ensure that all perspectives are heard.
- Don't be afraid of asking if you are not sure – ask respectfully without judgement.
- Don't be intimidated into avoiding difficult questions just because someone is from a visibly different background. It is worth remembering that all young people have an equal right in the UK to be heard and valued.
- Don't assume that because the last family from a similar background believed that mental illness is caused by spirits, for example, so will this family. There may be different factors at play.
- If there are a number of treatment options, don't assume what the family will choose. Discuss all the options and ensure the family are able to make an informed choice. Different families will need different levels of explanation and time.

Box 5.3 **Exercise**	• Reflect on how often you honestly consider the meaning of the material you cover with families. • How do you view culture and how it influences your practice?

A small-scale study found that Gujarati young people and their families valued professionals who were credible and respectful (Dogra *et al.* 2007). Having someone who was 'of the same ethnic background' was less of a preoccupation to them than it appears to service providers and policy-makers.

Mental state assessment

In younger children this will usually take the form of an observation of behaviour, particularly in relation to how they interact with their parents and siblings (if present). This may take the form of looking for normal developmental markers as well as social skills, appropriate eye contact, and danger signs such as 'frozen watchfulness'. In older children and young people this may be a much more formal process, looking at issues more familiar to a mental state examination in adults, such as:

- appearance – dress, gestures, posture, tics;
- mood – predominant feelings, lability of mood, fluctuations, appropriateness, ease or constriction of displaying feelings;
- manner of relating to the interviewer – perception and understanding of the process;
- modes of thinking and intellectual functioning;
- capacity for play and fantasy, amount and type of play, use of play materials, themes, spontaneity and interaction (after Johnson and Baggett 1995).

Observation of young people with their carers

While this may not be possible with some young people (e.g. in young people's services or substance misuse services, where young people may 'drop-in' for services or particularly wish their parents or carers not to be involved), it is usual to note the interactions between children, young people and their carers. This needs to be done in the context of what is appropriate for the child or young person's developmental stage, as outlined above. What is appropriate at a very young age may be interpreted as 'clinginess' for a slightly older child. Attachments to family and carers become looser in adolescents where part of the task is to develop appropriate levels of independence.

Risk assessment

The changing context

Risk management has become much more important in recent years with an increasingly litigious society. Within England, for example, provider Trusts contribute to the Clinical Negligence Scheme for Trusts, which is run by the National Health Servive (NHS) Litigation Authority, and is effectively an insurance scheme. Adherence to the published standards for risk management by Trusts means that they get a discount from their contributions. The standards vary slightly according to the nature of the Trust, but there are specific standards for mental health and learning disability Trusts (NHSLA 2008). These standards include the general principles of standardizing and measuring all forms of risk. There are also some medico-legal areas which require good governance of care provided, and while Subotsky (2003) discusses this from a medical point of view, the principles apply to all professional groups. The nature, source and assessment of the risks assessed should be recorded in a manner which is accessible to any staff likely to come into contact with the service user and their family. While these are general principles that could be applied to any form of risk management, there is also a growing tendency to codify these risks into a measurable score, and to standardize the manufacture of 'risk management plans'. It is important to recognize that CAMHS operates within a wider health care context, and should expect to adapt to wider health care community needs. While the need is clearer in adult settings (particularly in services which include crisis management teams and assertive outreach approaches) the measurement of risk is an important safeguard for both staff and service users. Within some areas of CAMHS practice, there are clear applications. These include self-harm (Anderson et al. 2004) and forensic areas (Tiffin and Kaplan 2004). In generic CAMHS the nature of the risk is slightly different, in that almost all the young people seen in specialist mental health services will have an adult with parental responsibility for the service user, and effectively they carry some of the responsibility for managing the risk associated with that child. This is somewhat different from more individually focused adult services, where the individual autonomy of service users, as fully grown adults, means that the risks associated with those service users are likely to be higher. For example, a young person who has self-harmed by overdosing on analgesics may well still be living with their parents. Any risk management plan associated with preventing further occurrences of self-harm is likely therefore to involve the parent(s), for example in monitoring availability of analgesics or other medications within the home. There may well be a number of complicating factors within the relationship to take into account, but the presence of a responsible adult in the house gives a different dimension to the management of risk, compared to a 35-year-old person living alone who suffers from depression.

Different aspects of risk

Risk has to be seen through several perspectives – risk to self and/or risk to others. There is the additional issue in children's services that all professionals who work with children have a responsibility to ensure they comply with local safeguarding procedures, as discussed below. Within CAMHS, therefore, there are areas where risk management is more important as a specific approach, and some areas where the parental system can largely be used as a way of ensuring risk is managed. There are also areas, however, where the parental system might be part of the problem, and the risk of child abuse through neglect or malice should also be considered. Often a good risk management plan will include the need to follow, or be aware of, child protection procedures. Other areas where risk management is of value are where young people are living independently of parental systems, or have very limited supervision of their lives. In these circumstances the need for an understanding of what support systems do exist, either formal or informal, is as important as it is in the case of adult treatment. The other main value of risk management procedures is in highlighting an element of the overall assessment which a clinician may well be conducting, but picking out and systematically recording those elements which indicate risk to self, to others or to staff.

Tools for risk assessment

Within a formal health care system, as we noted earlier, there may well be a systematic way of undertaking an assessment. Some health care providers will choose to develop their own risk management tools, while others will opt for a licensed and commercially available tool. One example of a commercial tool is the FACE risk profile. This is a licensed tool and should only be used if the licence is paid for by the employing health care provider. As an example of what risk profiles might include it is worth taking a look at the version that is available online at www.facecode.com. The risk profile uses a standardized (and validated) scoring system to high-light levels of risk in a simple numerical way, and then allows that risk to be quantified as a series of definitions. The profile then encourages recording of some of the most important elements of the risk, as assessed by the clinician, and some recording of the service users' own thoughts and perceptions of the risk. The final area allows for recording of a risk management plan. There is a temptation with any form to see it as a 'tick-box' approach, but it is not really possible to approach this area in such a simplistic way. What a risk management profile ought to allow is a distillation of a much wider assessment by a well-trained and experienced clinician, using all the skills they have learnt. All the information contained in a risk profile ought to be available elsewhere in the notes, recorded as part of the wider assessment. Some health care providers will, for example, use a particular colour of paper for the risk profile, and ensure that no other record within the case file is in that (often quite bright!) colour. This allows quick access to the most vital information in the event of a crisis. This can be further augmented, where electronic records are available, by the use of alert systems to collate such information into easily accessible areas such as the front page of an electronic record.

Box 5.4 Key components of a risk assessment

- Risk to self (from self or others).
- Risk to others.
- Awareness of risk.

Safeguarding children

This used be known as 'child protection' and over the last 20 years has become increasingly complex. Section 11 of the Children Act 2004 places a statutory duty on key people and bodies to make arrangements to safeguard and promote the welfare of children. Revised statutory guidance on the duty was issued in April 2007, however, safeguarding children has always been an issue that child mental health practitioners need to take into account as they assess children and their families. *Working Together to Safeguard Children* (HM Government 2006) sets out how individuals and organizations should work together to safeguard and promote the welfare of children. The guidance is addressed to all practitioners and front-line managers who have particular responsibilities for safeguarding and promoting the welfare of children, and to senior and operational managers in organizations that are responsible for commissioning or providing services to children, young people, parents and carers.

When undertaking a child mental assessment and when managing children with mental health problems, CAMHS nurses and other mental health clinicians have to be aware of the possibility of threats to children's physical and emotional safety. If as a nurse you have any concerns these need to be discussed with your supervisor and/or the safeguarding lead at your organization. It is rarely appropriate for mental health professionals to take the lead into investigating concerns. We do not propose to deal with this in any further detail but would just advise you to be aware of this issue (Powell 2007).

A specific nursing model for assessment: the Calgary Family Assessment and Intervention model

The Calgary Family Assessment and Intervention model is a useful way of amalgamating nursing theory and practice with a clear use of systemic ideas. Wright and Leahey (2000) have developed this model through three editions of their book *Nurses and Families*. The model is clear in its identification of its theoretical underpinnings, citing systemic theory, cybernetics communication and change theory. It also makes a strong argument for why it is a nursing intervention, and the role the nurse plays in making a change within a family system. As such the Calgary model falls within a structural or strategic family therapy approach, where there are clear attempts made to alter elements within the dynamics of a family system in the belief that a change in one part of the system will result in changes to other parts of the system (in this case the family system, with a corresponding therapeutic effect). Similarly, this model is very clear in describing how different concepts (such as family life cycles) can be used to practical effect, and it is this pragmatic approach which will appeal to nurses. In describing both the family assessment and family intervention elements of family systems nursing, great effort is made to outline in detail both the practical application and the theoretical thinking behind these actions in a way that will make sense to both nurses and family members. There is even a recognition of time pressures, and a description of how to fit the basic elements into a 'Fifteen Minute (or Shorter) Family Interview'. The way in which Wright and Leahey describe family systems nursing, and the Calgary model in particular, is attractive because of its understandability and pragmatic approach. While it acknowledges, for example, a debt to postmodernism in its understanding of the world, it has not gone on, as has much current systemic psychotherapy, to develop narrative approaches to change where the direct application to day-to-day life can be much harder to detect. The approach has also spawned a variety of literature which compares and contrasts it to other nursing models (such as Neuman's Systems Model, the Roy Adaptation Model, and the influence of Peplau on systemic approaches). Some of the most influential of these articles have been edited into a convenient single volume, *Readings in Family Nursing* (Wegner and Alexander 1999).

Box 5.5 Example of a CAMHS nursing assessment

This is a very brief example to illustrate the points made in the chapter and is not intended to suggest a new model, or to be a template. Refer to your own Trust's guidelines on record-keeping.

Name: Emma Chisset   **d.o.b.** 30.02.95. (Age 14)

ID/NHS no: 1234-456-7890

Address: 123 High Street, Anytown, Rutland

Genogram:

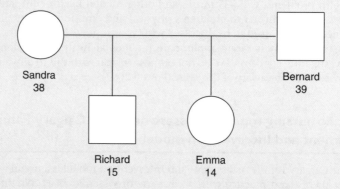

Presenting concerns

Emma has been feeling 'low' for several months, not wanting to go to school or to have contact with friends. She has been refusing to attend school for the last two weeks and becomes anxious and upset whenever the issue of school is brought up. She is an intelligent girl who had previously done well academically and had participated in organized activities, enjoyed swimming and been active.

Last week she confided to her mother that she felt life was not worth it, and that she had thought of throwing herself from a local bridge into the river. Mrs C immediately contacted her GP who referred Emma to CAMHS.

Family history

Parents have been together for nearly 20 years, married after living together for two years, and had their first child (Richard) soon after. They originally lived in Anytown (both parents were brought up there, and maternal grandparents still live there), but have moved around a lot over the last couple of years and this has involved the children moving schools on three occasions. This was because of Mr C's work commitments. The parents have realized the impact of the disruption on Emma and her sibling and have found work which will not involve any further moves for the immediate future.

Social history

Emma has had good peer relationships in the past, though these have been disrupted with the family moves. Although Emma had tried to keep in touch with friends via MSN and Facebook she has found it difficult to settle back to a peer group which has moved on while she was away from her home town.

Developmental history

Richard and Emma both walked and talked at 'normal times' according to their parents. Richard settled into nursery easily, though Emma was a little more 'clingy' and had some separation anxiety which settled after a few weeks. Emma had some problems with glue ear and needed grommets inserting, but this is now resolved.

Cultural issues

Bernard (Emma's father) is of Afro-Caribbean descent, while Sandra is white British. The family have good connections with the local Afro-Caribbean community and attend a Gospel Church. Emma and Richard have experienced some racist comments on the street (they live in a predominantly white area) but school has a mixed ethnic population and deals well, according to parents, with reported issues of bullying, particularly if there is an element of racially-based abuse.

Mental state

Emma presented as initially quite withdrawn, but responded to direct questions and gave good eye contact as the session progressed. She was able to concentrate well on what was asked of her and was spontaneous in correcting things that her brother said which she disagreed with. She was well dressed and her parents did not report any concerns about her ability to continue to look after herself. Emma said that although she felt low most of the time she had only briefly thought of killing herself and felt better for sharing this with her mother. She has not self-harmed and described feeling rather frightened by the thoughts. There was no planning towards suicide and she denied feeling actively like she wanted to hurt herself or end her life now.

Observation of interactions

Emma sat next to her mother and was initially reluctant to answer questions. She responded well to her father gently explaining the importance of her answering honestly so that the nurse could understand how she felt and help her. Interactions with her brother were mostly to correct things he said with which she disagreed.

Risk assessment

Emma has had thoughts of harming herself but denies these currently.

She has agreed that if she has a recurrence of these thoughts she will talk to her mother again, and demonstrates enough insight that the family feel she will be able to do this.

If her mother is not available she felt she could talk to her father (but not her brother), or would text her mother if she was at work.

Risk Level 2
Formulation

Emma presents as having a moderate level of depression, probably resulting from repeated moves of house and school, and loss of peer group.

No current suicidal ideation, but has had thoughts of self-harm which may recur, and for which there is a plan which Emma feels she can use to gain support.

Care plan

- Family sessions to ensure that the family understand Emma's feelings and can support her.
- Individual sessions for Emma to explore how she feels and be able to articulate those feelings.
- Contact education welfare service to look at getting school work to do at home, and begin looking at reintegration into school.
- Briefly explain importance of good diet and exercise in maintaining good mental health.
- Continue assessment of low mood and consider getting Emma seen by a child psychiatrist if mood does not lift.

Signed: A. Nurse   Clinical Nurse Specialist   Date: 31/03/09

Summary

Assessment takes many forms, depending on the role and function of the nurse at any given time. This chapter has highlighted some areas which are particularly important in CAMHS, and made one suggestion for a specific nursing model of family care which can be used in CAMHS. We have also focused on areas such as development and culture which are important but in practice are often covered less well than other aspects.

References

AAMC (Association of American Medical Colleges) (1999) Report III: contemporary issues, in *Medicine, Communication in Medicine: Spirituality, Cultural Issues and End of Life Care*, Medical School Objectives Project. Washington, DC: AAMC.

Altschul, A.T. (1972) *Patient-Nurse Interaction: A Study of Interactive Patterns on Adult Psychiatric Wards*. Edinburgh: Churchill Livingstone.

Anderson, L., Scrimshaw. S., Fullilove, M., Fielding. J., Normand. J. and The Task Force on Community

Preventive Services (2003) Culturally competent healthcare systems: a systematic review, *American Journal of Preventative Medicine*, 24(3S): 68–79.

Anderson, M., Woodward, L. and Armstrong, M. (2004) Self-harm in young people: a perspective for mental health care, *International Nursing Review*, 51(4): 222–8.

Barker, P. (1999) *The Philosophy and Practice of Psychiatric Nursing*. London: Churchill Livingstone.

Bennett, J., Kalathil, J. and Keating, F. (2007) *Race Equality Training in Mental Health Services in England: Does One Size Fit All?* London: The Sainsbury Centre for Mental Health.

Bolton, P. (2001) Developmental assessment, *Advances in Psychiatric Treatment*, 7: 32–42.

Brown, B., Crawford, P. and Carter, R. (2006) *Evidence-based Health Communication*. Maidenhead: Open University Press.

Dogra, N. (2003) Cultural competence or cultural sensibility? A comparison of two ideal type models to teach cultural diversity to medical students, *International Journal of Medicine*, 5(4): 223–31.

Dogra, N. and Karim, K. (2005) Training in diversity for psychiatrists, *Advances in Psychiatric Treatment*, 11: 159–67.

Dogra, N., Vostanis, P., Abuateya, H. and Jewson, N. (2007) Children's mental health services and ethnic diversity: Gujarati families' perspectives of service provision for mental health problems, *Transcultural Psychiatry*, 44(2): 275–91.

Dugdale, A.E. and Chen, S.T. (1979) Ethnic differences in the Goodenough-Harris draw a man and draw a woman tests, *Archives of Diseases in Childhood*, 54(11): 880–5.

Evans, M. (1999) Nursing care for children and adolescents with mental health disorders, in M. Clinton and S. Nelson (eds) *Advanced Practice in Mental Health Nursing*. Oxford: Blackwell.

Goodenough, F.L. (1926) *Measurement of Intelligence by Drawings*. New York: World Book Company.

HM Government (2006) *Working Together to Safeguard Children: A Guide to Inter-agency Working to Safeguard and Promote the Welfare of Children*. London: TSO.

Johnson, B.S. and Baggett, J.M. (1995) Applying the nursing process to children, adolescents and families, in B.S. Johnson (ed.) *Child, Adolescent and Family Psychiatric Nursing*. Philadelphia, PA: J.B. Lippincott.

McDonald, L., Rennie, A., Tolmie, J., Galloway, P. and McWilliam, R. (2006) Investigation of global developmental delay, *Archives of Disease in Childhood*, 91: 701–5.

McDougall, T. (ed.) (2006) *Child and Adolescent Mental Health Nursing*. Oxford: Blackwell.

NHSLA (NHS Litigation Authority) (2008) *Risk Management Standards for Mental Health and Learning Disability Trusts*, www.nhsla.com/RiskManagement/CnstStandards/, accessed 24 November 2008.

Peplau, H. (1982) Interpersonal techniques: the crux of psychiatric nursing, in S. Smoyak and S. Rouslin (eds) *A Collection of Classics in Psychiatric Nursing Literature*. Thorofare, NJ: Charles B. Slack Inc.

Pillitteri, A. (2006) *Maternal and Child Health Nursing: Care of the Childbearing and Childrearing Family*, 5th edn. Philadephia, PA: Lippincott, Williams & Wilkins.

Powell, C. (2007) *Safeguarding Children and Young People: A Guide for Nurses and Midwives*. Maidenhead: Open University Press.

Sparrow, S., Balla, D. and Cicchetti, D. (2007) *Vineland Adaptive Behaviour Scales*, 2nd edn. Swindon: GL Assessment.

Subotsky, F. (2003) Clinical risk management and child mental health, *Advances in Psychiatric Treatment*, 9: 319–26.

Tiffin, P. and Kaplan, C. (2004) Dangerous children: assessment and management of risk, *Child and Adolescent Mental Health*, 9(2): 56–64.

Wegner, G.D. and Alexander, R.J. (1999) *Readings in Family Nursing*, 2nd edn. Philadelphia, PA: Lippincott, Williams & Wilkins.

Wright, L.M. and Leahey, M. (2000) *Nurses and Families: A Guide to Family Assessment and Intervention*, 3rd edn. Philadelphia, PA: F.A. Davis.

Further reading

Dogra, N., Vostanis, P., Abuateya, H. and Jewson, N. (2005) Understanding of mental health and mental illness by Gujarati young people and their parents, *Diversity in Health and Social Care*, 8: 91–8.

Dogra, N., Vostanis, P. and Karnik, N. (2007) Child and adolescent psychiatric disorders, in D. Bhugra and K. Bhui (eds) *Textbook of Cultural Psychiatry*. Cambridge: Cambridge University Press.

Karnik, N., Dogra, N. and Vostanis, P. (2007) The management of child and adolescent psychiatric disorders, in D. Bhugra and K. Bhui (eds) *Textbook of Cultural Psychiatry*. Cambridge: Cambridge University Press.

Powell, C. (2007) *Safeguarding Children and Young People: A Guide for Nurses and Midwives*. Maidenhead: Open University Press.

6 | Counselling and the therapeutic use of self

Sharon Leighton

> I keep six honest serving men
> (They taught me all I knew)
> Their names are What and Why and When
> And How and Where and Who.
>
> (Kipling 1902)[1]

Key features	
	• Provides a framework for discussing counselling in child and adolescent mental health services (CAMHS).
	• Explores the therapeutic use of self.
	• Highlights core counselling skills.
	• Reviews three models of counselling.

Introduction

Counselling remains an ambiguous and much used term, with no single, consensually agreed definition to date. The term is also frequently used interchangeably with psychotherapy. Broadly, it involves an agreement between two parties to work together in trying to understand and resolve certain psychological difficulties held by one of them. However, a distinction needs to be made between the informed and informal use of such skills and the possession of accredited qualifications in psychotherapy and/or counselling.

In the introduction to this book we identify that nursing is both an art and a science. This chapter provides an example of combining the two elements. We begin by exploring the therapeutic use of self. Core generic counselling skills are then defined, and these skills are subsequently taken one stage further through discussing three different paradigms that emphasize the therapeutic use of self – i.e. person-centred, psychodynamic and integrative approaches. The choice of models is based on the fact that the first two approaches have greatly influenced the development of many other models.[2] The final section is a case study, relating theory to practice. Although the therapeutic use of self and counselling skills are considered separately for ease of discussion, they overlap and are inevitably interlinked. The significance of counselling skills for CAMH nurses working across the tiers is demonstrated through the discussion.

Although the need for regular clinical supervision is highlighted, it is not discussed in depth; its importance is evident throughout the discussion. Similarly, the significance of practical

---

[1] Kipling, R. (1902) The Elephant's Child, from the *Just So Stories*. This can be a useful quote in terms of encouraging reflection on what we are doing and why.

[2] Family therapy and cognitive-behavioural approaches are discussed in Chapters 7 and 8 respectively.

issues such as time-keeping, contracting and note-taking is taken as read and not discussed here. The importance of developmental consideration is noted (developmental issues are the focus of Chapter 2). The generic terms 'practitioner' and 'client' are used to refer to counsellor/ therapist/nurse or children, young people and their families respectively.

The final points to highlight are that while many adolescents and most adults seek counselling of their own volition, children are usually brought by parents or other significant adults, who may have their own agenda. Furthermore, however much an approach advocates helping clients to help themselves, there are times when practitioners working in CAMHS have to take action to safeguard children.

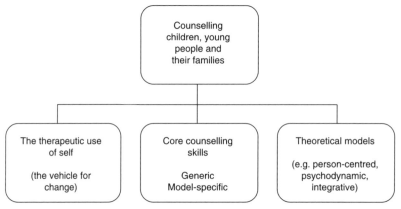

Figure 6.1 A framework for discussing counselling in CAMHS

The therapeutic use of self

An integral part of the therapeutic use of self is caring about what we are doing – i.e. being able to hold the client(s) in mind; creating the mental space with them to facilitate change and growth. Caring about what we are doing enables us to do it skilfully – i.e. to combine art and science. However, the therapeutic use of self is influenced by contextual factors, including external and organizational pressures, personal 'life' issues (e.g. illness in a family member), competence and confidence.

In this section three questions are explored:

- What is the nature of the therapeutic relationship?
- What is the purpose of the therapeutic relationship?
- What makes a successful therapeutic relationship?

The nature of the therapeutic relationship

The therapeutic relationship has long been recognized as a key factor in successful therapy with adults. Different orientations use similar terms (e.g. empathy) when discussing qualities associated with the therapeutic relationship, and also very diverse ones:

- person-centred: genuineness, non-possessive warmth, self-disclosure;
- psychodynamic: counter-transference, projective identification (Rowan and Jacobs 2008).

These terms are discussed later in the section on theoretical models.

A good therapeutic relationship contains variables common to different clinical orientations. These include empathy, warmth, acceptance and encouragement of risk-taking, with mutual trust and confidence characterizing the relationship (Salzberger 1970; Austen 2000; Asay and Lambert 2001; Jacobs 2004; Mearns and Thorne 2007). In a study of Australian adolescent inpatient units, the nature of the therapeutic relationship that developed between nurses and adolescents was characterized as engaged, relational, mutual, informed and ethical (Geanellos 2002). For children accessing CAMHS the ideal helpful professional is perceived as empathic, emotionally available, trustworthy, understanding and able to make things happen (Farnfield and Kaszap 1998).

Therapeutic work with children and their families occurs within an interpersonal context. Asay and Lambert (2001) argue that there is substantial evidence indicating that the quality of the therapeutic relationship has a large influence on the success of any interventions with children and families. As the interpersonal context transcends families, good inter-agency relationships are also deemed essential (Urwin 2007). However, in their review of existing findings regarding the 'youth working alliance'[3] Zack et al. (2007) identify that there is no single definition of the 'youth working alliance', thus making it difficult to assess research results. They also identify that the therapeutic relationship is affected by several patient and therapist characteristics – example 1: an anxious child is more likely to work at developing relationships than a more antisocial child; example 2: the interpersonal skills of the therapist (e.g. empathy, warmth, genuineness) have a positive effect on the relationship. It is essential to further our understanding of the nature of the therapeutic relationship through research into how family systems affect attendance and the development of the relationship, how child development may affect their ability to form therapeutic relationships, and the effects of adolescent development on forming and maintaining the relationship (Zack et al. 2007).

The purpose of the therapeutic relationship

The therapeutic relationship can be seen as a vehicle for inspiring hope and nurturing the development of coping skills.

The interpersonal relationship is, in and of itself, an intervention for inspiring hope in people with mental health problems (Peplau 1988). Koehn and Cutcliffe (2007) undertook a systematic review of the mental health nursing literature that focuses on inspiring hope within a counselling relationship (three related to adolescents). Findings show consistently that the therapeutic relationship acts as a conduit for the generation of hope.

Nurses work toward fostering developmental skills such as independence in adolescents and functional coping skills for dealing with distress and challenging behaviour in personal, interpersonal and social contexts (Geanellos 2002).

Developing a successful therapeutic relationship

A successful therapeutic relationship requires both the utilization of skills and the therapeutic use of self. Skill employment and the therapeutic use of self require the mental space to be able to hold the client(s) in mind. It is this aspect which is addressed first.

---

[3] The term 'working alliance' is used in psychodynamic theory to refer to the therapeutic relationship. In this chapter the latter term is used.

Creating space and holding in mind

Having the space to hold the client in mind and providing them with the mental space to address their concerns is central to the therapeutic relationship. Brazier (2001) emphasizes the importance of listening, of creating space for the client to be heard. He suggests that 'therapy begins with cleaning up the space inside ourselves' (p. 32). He emphasizes that listening unconditionally for an hour is difficult unless the practitioner has learnt to quieten their mind and listen. Therefore, it is essential that we create the mental space to *hear* others and help them to create their own space in which to begin to address their difficulties. In order to be able to use the self therapeutically, it is essential to create the mental space to be able to hold the client in mind and to be able to recognize what is being communicated non-verbally – for example, an adolescent might say 'don't let's go there', when a question is posed, but the anguish behind the quickly spoken words that is evident in the tone used and the momentary look of pain could easily be missed if the practitioner does not have the mental space to listen and hear.

Box 6.1	• What helps you in creating and nurturing your own mental space?
Exercise	

Having the mental space, individually and as a team, enables practitioners to think about and make sense of what is happening in each situation. Furthermore, it provides a 'temporary secure base' from which young people in crisis and their families can safely explore and grow (Bowley and Bratley 2005). A sense of mental space is also important for processing the changes and difficulties faced by adolescents, as these often involve intense feelings. The worker's capacity to think can be undermined by the anxiety projected by the adolescent. It is important to find a space in the mind when thinking about feelings in order to contain the adolescent's distress and disturbance. For the adolescent, being kept in mind is important for developing their own mental space; if there is space in someone else's mind, it is possible to have the notion of space in one's own mind (Bowley and Baratley 2005).

Having the mental space to think and reflect on the feelings and ideas evoked in us through contact with another person is an increasing challenge in the current target-driven culture that prevails in health and social care. In this climate there is often considerable pressure to act or 'do' something. This poses ethical dilemmas as well as frustration and increased risk to children, adolescents and their families.

Box 6.2	• How often have you heard a colleague utter the words, 'I don't have the space to think about this child and their family'?
Exercise	• What do you think are the potential implications for the practitioner, and the children and families with whom they are working when this is the situation?
	• Think of two cases – one where you had the mental space to listen, hear and reflect and one where you didn't. Where there any differences in the process and/or the outcome?

Skills

Skills are discussed at length in the next section. Suffice it is to say here that those necessary for a successful therapeutic relationship include self-awareness, communication and listening skills, reflective practice, and knowledge and understanding of different developmental levels and associated ways of communicating.

Self-awareness involves knowing our own values and beliefs and how these influence attitudes and behaviour. It incorporates the ability to see oneself as others may. It includes the ability to reflect on the process if, for example, an interaction with a young person arouses strong feelings.

Box 6.3
Exercise
- Reflect on how anxiety may affect people's attitudes and behaviour.
- Identify potential sources of anxiety in your work with children, adolescents and their families.
- Reflect on ways in which you might tackle anxiety associated with:
  - the young person;
  - own knowledge and skills;
  - support and links with others;
  - individual issues.

Therapeutic use of self

The practitioner embodies the essence of counselling (Brazier 2001; Mearns and Thorne 2007; Rowan and Jacobs 2008). The use of self is both covert (through self-monitoring and the development of inner attitudes and aptitudes) and overt (through disclosure). The practitioner's use of self is what distinguishes those who have learnt the skills of a theoretical model from those who have moved beyond dependence upon skills to a greater use of themselves in the therapeutic relationship; there is a readiness to relate person-to-person alongside their skills. Consideration is not only given to the feelings that the client engenders in the practitioner, but also to how the practitioner uses their cognitive, emotional and intuitive responses, whatever their origin (Rowan and Jacobs 2008).

Creating the mental space identified earlier can be seen as starting with the therapist. Rogers' (1967) conditions of empathy, unconditional appreciation and genuineness play a vital role in being with another person in such a way that frees them to face their emotional turmoil. From a person-centred perspective the emphasis is on involvement, intimacy and emotional risk (Mearns and Thorne 2007). However, such an approach runs counter to much in the prevailing culture. For many in the helping professions the current climate, fostered by much recent legislation, encourages an attitude of caution and fearfulness which leads to a culpable under-involvement with those who are often in most need of assistance (e.g. young people who are depressed and possibly suicidal). This creates a continual uncomfortable dissonance for the person-centred counsellor working in the health service or in education, both heavily controlled by social control politics. The irony here is that professionals in both sectors are fundamentally concerned with the whole person and their development (Mearns and Thorne 2007).

From a psycho-dynamic perspective, attitudes which foster perceptiveness and therapeutic interaction include the practitioner's attitude towards the client. An appropriate attitude includes (Salzberger 1970):

- open-mindedness;
- curiosity;

- attending to verbal and non-verbal communication;
- listening and waiting;
- taking feelings seriously;
- understanding, holding and containing mental pain.

Box 6.4   • Consider the similarities and differences between the two approaches. Are the
Exercise   differences more than just semantics?

The next section focuses on core counselling skills.

Core counselling skills

There are numerous textbooks providing in-depth theoretical and practical explanations about counselling skills. Here the focus is on highlighting the core skills identified by Culley and Bond (2004) and Inskipp (2006). These skills are perceived as transcending theoretical orientation, although this is yet to be proven. Moreover, the three core *Rogerian* qualities of empathic understanding, unconditional positive regard and congruence are seen as central to any counselling endeavour.

Inskipp (2006) identifies the inner and outer skills necessary to achieve this. Inner skills refer to inside awareness/process skills, while outer skills refer to those that can be seen and evaluated by an observer. Inner skills include:

- observing;
- listening;
- body scanning for awareness of body sensations, emotions, thoughts and images;
- impartial witnessing;
- discriminating;
- reflecting.

Outer skills include:

- attending;
- greeting;
- active listening: paraphrasing, reflecting feelings, summarizing;
- asking questions;
- contracting: purpose stating, preference stating;
- clarifying (the therapeutic) role;
- technical skills (e.g. recording a session).

Inskipp suggests that in order to learn and practise these skills it is necessary to break each one down into smaller elements. For example, contracting involves negotiating, which, in turn, involves the micro-skills of listening, paraphrasing and reflecting feelings. It is these specific micro skills that can be identified, practised, internalized and developed into the practitioner's way of working. These micro-skills can be seen as synonymous with the core skills identified by Culley and Bond (2004):

- active listening;
- reflective skills;
- probing skills.

These are expanded on briefly here in order to demonstrate how they underpin different approaches.

Active listening involves listening purposefully and responding in such a way that clients recognize that they have been both heard and understood. It involves both attending and listening. Attending acts as a basis for listening to and observing clients. It is a way of giving clients your presence (i.e. 'holding them in mind'). Attending well conveys acceptance, understanding and genuineness.

Adopting a receptive attitude involves taking account of and thinking about feelings and ideas evoked in ourselves on the basis of our contact with another person. It involves pausing for thought or finding some space to think when there might be considerable pressure to act or 'do' something. It fosters understanding of what is happening in the session and for the client.

Some of the major barriers to active listening are associated with:

- culture;
- personal values;
- issues in the practitioner's own life (Culley and Bond 2004).

In addition there is the issue of practitioners working under pressure (mentioned previously), so that they do not have the mental space to hear what is being said (verbally and non-verbally) and what is left unsaid.

Reflective and probing skills are used to respond verbally to a client. Reflective skills are verbal skills which a practitioner uses in order to demonstrate that they have an understanding of what the client is telling them. They are powerful skills for both building a therapeutic relationship and obtaining information. Reflective skills are:

- restating what is perceived as a significant word or phrase;
- paraphrasing – i.e. conveying the client's central message, using your own words; accurate paraphrasing is essential for communicating empathic understanding and for relationship-building;
- summarizing, offering a précis of important themes or concerns (Culley and Bond 2004).

Probing is an important aspect of the counselling process as there will be times when the practitioner may want to influence the direction of exploration. However, care is urged when using these skills as they can be experienced as intrusive. Probing skills include:

- questioning;
- making statements (Culley and Bond 2004).

Questions can both facilitate and inhibit exploration. Open questions (e.g. 'What usually happens when . . .?' are more likely to generate discussion than questions requiring a 'yes/no' or 'either/or' response. Hypothetical questions are useful for helping clients to articulate and explore feelings and consider alternative outcomes (e.g. 'What do you imagine would happen if you were to say no to her?')

Making statements is a mild form of probing; statements tend to be less intrusive and controlling than questions (e.g. 'You have explained how you and your husband respond very differently to Jake's tantrums. I wonder how that makes you feel').

Finally, it has been suggested that training needs to focus on facilitating the development and monitoring of the skills of self-awareness (see Box 6.5), rather than solely on teaching specific communication skills. The justification for this is that while skills can be learnt, practised and used as 'techniques', their therapeutic use depends on both the communication skills, and the attitude and intention of the practitioner. In order for practice to have a genuine and helpful impact, feelings, insight and knowledge need to be recognized and articulated. Furthermore, the way in which information is communicated is central to the process. Therefore, a competent practitioner is someone who is skilled in interpersonal communication, can establish and maintain relationships, and who is self-aware (Culley and Bond 2004; Inskipp 2006) – one who is skilled in the therapeutic use of self.

Box 6.5 Self-awareness

Self-awareness involves:

- knowing our own values and beliefs and how these influence our attitudes and behaviour;
- the ability to see ourselves as others may;
- the ability to reflect on the process – for example, noticing when interaction with a young person arouses strong feelings and our reaction to these feelings.

The core skills discussed can be seen as integral to the therapeutic models reviewed in the next section.

Theoretical models of counselling

It can be helpful to view theory as a working conceptual model for understanding and making sense of experience. The underlying principles of three different approaches form the basis of this section. The theoretical frameworks reviewed here are:

- person-centred;
- psycho-dynamic;
- integrative.

Person-centred counselling

While the theoretical underpinnings of the person-centred approach include an understanding of personality development and the therapeutic process, the initial concern for the counsellor is the understanding and valuing their own being – i.e. self-awareness and acceptance. The person-centred approach places great emphasis on the presence, authenticity, self-awareness and congruence of the practitioner. However, it is not only a case of the practitioner offering relational depth, the client responding, and the process being helpful. The key variable that will impact upon the client's changing is the client's *agency*; the extent of their ability to think, feel and act as an autonomous being who has the confidence to trust their own experience within the constraints of their social context (Mearns and Thorne 2007). Therefore, a central assumption of the person-centred approach is that the client can be trusted to find their own way forward if only the counsellor can be the kind of companion who is capable of encouraging a relationship where the client can begin to feel safe and to experience self-acceptance. The practitioner needs to adopt the three core conditions of the model when with the client, to enable the client's actualizing tendency to begin to work (Rogers 1951; Mearns and Thorne 2007).

The core conditions of the person-centred approach

The three 'core Rogerian conditions' are empathy, unconditional positive regard and genuineness (Rogers 1951; Mearns and Thorne 2007):

- *Empathy:* to feel and communicate a deep empathic understanding is not a 'technique' used to respond to the client, but a *way-of-being-in-relation-to* the client; the humanity of the counsellor reaching out, not just to one part, but to the whole humanity of their client. Where there is *empathic understanding*, the counsellor demonstrates a capacity to track and sense accurately the feelings and personal meanings of the client; they are able to discover what it feels like to be that client in that situation and to perceive the world as the client does. Furthermore, they develop the ability to communicate to the client this sensitive and acceptant understanding.
- *Unconditional positive regard:* therapeutic movement is more likely to occur when a counsellor is able to embrace an attitude of acceptance and non-judgementalism. The counsellor's acceptance enables the client to feel safe to begin exploring negative feelings and to move into the heart of their angst. It also easier to face one's self more honestly without an ever present fear of rejection or condemnation.
- *Genuineness:* the more the counsellor is able to be themselves in the relationship without putting up a professional or personal facade, the greater will be the chance of the client changing and developing in a positive and constructive manner. This includes being transparent and a refusal to encourage an image of being superior or expert. A counsellor who is congruent conveys the message that it is not only permissible but desirable to be oneself. In such a relationship the client is more likely to find inner resources and not cling to any expectation that the counsellor will provide the answers for them.

These core conditions represent the central dimensions of the therapeutic relationship. All three operate in unison; it is not therapeutic to be genuine if the practitioner has neither empathy nor positive regard.

Box 6.6 **Exercise**	• When might a person-centred approach be useful with a young person? • What might be some of the challenges involved in adopting the three core conditions? How might these be addressed?

Psycho-dynamic counselling

This model incorporates psycho-dynamic understanding of personal development and of internal relations within the psyche. It is recognized that the client's past experience can inform the present situation and that the present situation colours their memories of the past. The individual's personal history has a significant influence on the relationship between practitioner and client (Jacobs 2004).

A psychodynamic approach depends on the client's ability to communicate through words (or play in the case of children) and feelings, without acting out;[4] an ability to listen, reflect on, respond to, agree with and, if necessary, contradict the practitioner; the ability to form their

---

[4] That is, expressing unconscious feelings and fantasies in behaviour; reacting to present situations as if they were the original situation that gave rise to the feelings and fantasies.

own ideas, outside sessions as well as within them, demonstrating a wish to understand, and so share responsibility for finding answers with the therapist (Jacobs 2004).

This approach involves finely balancing a number of ways of being with the client: firstly, holding back in order to allow the client space to develop their own story and associations, and to discover where a practitioner's own feelings and reactions throw light on the interpersonal relationship. Secondly, encouraging the client to reflect on what they are saying and feeling, sometimes following a lead. Thirdly, being genuine, and not allowing the counselling role to become a mask for ordinary human responses and reactions (Salzberger 1970; Urwin 2003; Jacobs 2004).

Providing space and containing mental pain

Within this model clients are provided with a setting where they are both listened to, and able to listen to their own thoughts, explore feelings and look for clues. A practitioner, by acting as a container for the fears associated with this task, and showing by their attitude that they are not 'all knowing' either, makes it possible for a client to accomplish a task which they could not accomplish on their own (Salzberger 1970; Hunter 2001).

Within a psycho-dynamic approach the practitioner adopts a receptive attitude that enables them to take in the appearance of the client (e.g. dress as well as body language), what is said verbally and expressed non-verbally, the mood and feelings communicated, and to be aware of feelings and ideas evoked in the practitioner on the basis of what the client is communicating: 'Being receptive means using one's mind as an instrument sensitive to the vibrations and echoes set off in it by someone else's projections' (Salzberger 1970: 138).

A dynamic process occurs when a receptive person is able to listen, understand and contain mental pain. The client, finding their feelings of anxiety, aggression and despair accepted and contained, is enabled, at a feeling level, to realize that someone is capable of living with the feared or rejected aspect of themselves. The experience of having these feelings accepted and contained enables the client to think about, clarify, differentiate, give a vague feeling a name and link it to what is meaningful, and so transform pain (Salzberger 1970; Hunter 2001).

This process of projective identification involves either communicating or disposing of an unwanted part of the personality (e.g. pressing unwanted feelings out of one's mind and into someone else), so that someone else can bear those feelings with, or for, them – for example, experiencing the sense of pure desolation in a bereaved adolescent who sits silently in a session. Salzberger (1970) suggests that the theory of projective identification, and our susceptibility to penetration by another person's mental pain, gives this experience depth and purpose, as well as explaining its therapeutic importance. This kind of communication is often non-verbal, accompanying, and sometimes contradicting, what is consciously communicated (Salzberger 1970). For example, a parent might speak in a matter-of-fact manner about the death of a grandparent three years ago while projecting a sense of deep sorrow. A practitioner's ability to be receptive depends on their being in touch with feelings (i.e. self-aware).

Transference and counter-transference

Although the psycho-dynamic practitioner will ultimately be judged by the quality of the therapeutic relationship, this is not primarily what psycho-dynamic counselling is about. Jacobs (2004) considers that psycho-dynamic counselling goes beyond the core conditions identified by person-centred practitioners. He argues that it provides a fuller picture with which to understand the different dimensions of the therapeutic relationship. These dimensions include the emphasis on transference and counter-transference. The therapeutic relationship (like any relationship) can equally be influenced by transference reactions on the part of the client, or by counter-transference reactions on the part of the practitioner. In this context, transference refers to the redirection of a client's feelings from a significant person in their life to the therapist (e.g. feelings of rage associated with a parent). Counter-transference refers to the redirection of a therapist's feelings toward a client, or to unconscious or instinctive emotion felt towards the client. A therapist's attunement to their own counter-transference is nearly as critical as their understanding of the transference (Jacobs 2004).

The focus in psycho-dynamic counselling is, largely, the practitioner and the client recognizing the transference relationship and exploring what the meaning of that relationship is. Feelings and ideas that the client has about counselling seen in the transference aspect of their relationship can reveal feelings and ideas present in past and current relationships. Through resolving the transference, it is possible to rework some past experiences and current relationships (Jacobs 2004).

Integrative counselling approaches

Geldard and Geldard (2006) suggest that while there are several different approaches to counselling children, it is usually advantageous to use an integrative model where strategies from different therapeutic approaches are used at particular points in the therapeutic process. This enables the counsellor to work with the wider system (e.g. parents/carers, school) and to work individually with the child where necessary, using different and developmentally appropriate media and activities.

Horton (2006) identifies that over time most counsellors tend gradually to develop their own individual styles of working, using a conceptual framework based on more than one theoretical model. This integration is differentiated from an eclectic approach, which is viewed as more of a random ad hoc process. There is no one approach to integrative counselling. Currently there is little objective and empirical research to support the effectiveness of such models. Reasons for this include methodological problems associated with measuring personal and individual combinations of ideas and methods (Horton 2006). Here the model discussed is *integrated* eclecticism.

Integrated eclecticism: a therapeutic synthesis

Eclecticism draws on many different theoretical approaches that embrace differing beliefs and assumptions concerning human nature. An integrated eclecticism (in contrast to an unplanned, ad hoc approach) requires a model which maintains a theoretical coherence and posits specific principles of application (Austen 2000).

The underlying theoretical framework of the model is based on systems theory; clients are viewed not only as interactive parts of wider systems (e.g. families), but also as having systems within themselves (i.e. internal, interactive psychological systems of cognition, affect and behaviour). The framework incorporates various approaches including family therapy, cognitive behavioural therapy (CBT), existential and psycho-dynamic models. In an integrative approach, theory is explained in terms of circular rather than linear causality (Austen 2000).

Austen (2000) asserts that:

- clients pass through similar stages of conceptual organization in all psychological therapies;
- different therapies focus on different levels of awareness in the reorganization process;
- different therapies work to bring about different levels of change.

Based on these assumptions, she argues that the therapy of choice can be chosen by identifying at what level change is required and by assessing the client's level of processing of the problematic experience. 'First order' change aims to increase understanding and communication within relationships and/or to bring about behavioural change, rather than to promote profound change in underlying mental structures. Indicators for first order change requiring a systemic change include a problem defined as in a relationship – for example, where a young person is returning home from care. Approaches used at this level are either behavioural or family therapy. Should second order change be indicated, an assessment is made of the client's conceptualization of the problem in order to define the treatment strategy. Clients with warded off, painful feelings indicate a psycho-dynamic approach, clients showing vague awareness an existential approach, and those showing a clear conceptualization of the problem a CBT approach.

Further assessment is an interactive, evolving process that allows for a change in therapeutic orientation as the therapy progresses. Therefore, it is possible to adapt the approach as necessary and to move between approaches as required (Austen 2000).

The therapeutic relationship lies at the heart of this model. It requires great sensitivity on the part of the practitioner – first to assess the client's readiness in terms of the assimilation continuum; second, to move to a different approach if required (and the client is comfortable with this). The therapeutic relationship always takes priority. A change in approach is not to suggest a change in the practitioner's *being* with the client, but rather that the therapeutic approach utilized may be informed by different therapeutic approaches. It is a case of working within the overall framework of the model while maintaining the therapeutic relationship (Austen 2000).

In summary, similarities between the approaches include that all:

- are non-intrusive and give the client considerable freedom;
- use the therapeutic relationship as a vehicle for change;
- emphasize the importance of creating space to enable the client to progress;
- create space through the therapeutic use of self;
- consider the development of practitioner self-awareness as vital to the process.

In the case study presented next, an integrative approach is used. Within the context of the therapeutic relationship the case study draws upon the author's knowledge of bereavement, developmental and systems theory and, as Ben and his mother had an awareness of what was wrong at an existential level, uses a person-centred approach.

Box 6.7 Case scenario: Ben's story[5]

Ben Bentley, aged 12, was referred by his GP with behavioural problems, thought to be associated with the death of his father by suicide three years previously. I met with Ben and his mother together at the initial appointment as Ben did not want to be seen individually. The story that unfolded during the assessment session was as follows.

Ben lived with his mother and 14-year-old brother, Matthew. His father was described as having had a long history of depression associated with dislike of change, difficulty coping with stress and being very intense and possessive with his wife. He apparently sought psychiatric help on several occasions but Mrs Bentley felt that 'the system' failed him. Six months before Mr Bentley's death the marital relationship was reported to

---

[5] Both Ben and Mrs Bentley willingly gave their consent for me to share Ben's story. Their identities have been changed for reasons of confidentiality.

have been so strained that Mr Bentley began to sleep at the flat above his business. He is reported to have been increasingly angry and unhappy about all areas of his life. He strangled himself with a length of rope early one morning. There was no suicide note and the way that various things had been left suggested that this had been an impulsive act. Mrs Bentley and the boys had last seen Mr Bentley the previous lunchtime when he had appeared to be angry and upset and had left abruptly. They learnt of his death from the police 24 hours later.

Ben was described as being a child with a difficult/feisty temperament, but who had been lively and happy until his father's death when he was 9. Initially Ben had appeared to carry on as if nothing had happened. Mrs Bentley did not press information on him but waited for him to approach her before telling him things. On reflection she wished that she had told him earlier. Ben had only begun asking questions after 12–18 months and this had coincided with deterioration in his behaviour and peer relationships within school. Mrs Bentley felt that the attitudes of staff and pupils had made things very difficult for Ben in his last year at primary school. He had moved to a senior school in another catchment area shortly before I met with him. At that time he remained unsettled and socially isolated. At home he was described as unhappy, volatile and completely lacking in motivation. Ben reported that he had felt sad most of the time since his father died and angry all the time. He was easily irritated by trivial things, had very poor concentration and little enthusiasm for anything. His attitude was extremely negative most of the time. He argued constantly with his mother and was possessive with her. He had no sense of purpose in life and no hope for the future. He had major difficulties with sleep. His symptoms of depression appeared to be continuous and unrelenting. He denied any suicidal ideation.

In the session Ben was upset and tearful throughout and appeared to be depressed. My initial impression was of disabling grief with accompanying depression in a 12-year-old boy who had a difficult/feisty temperament and whose father had committed suicide three years previously.

I asked a psychiatrist colleague to assess Ben with a view to considering the use of antidepressant medication to lift his mood before starting therapy. At this stage it was decided that I would commence weekly grief therapy with Ben and medication would be considered in the future should Ben prove to be too low in mood to make use of the sessions or if there was no subsequent change in his mental state.

My role in the therapeutic process was to be a skilled companion on a journey where a new life story was created which enabled Ben (and his mother) to find new meaning through a process which involved them actively grieving for what they had lost, confronting their loss and attempting to understand it through self-reflection. With regard to both the session frequency and number, Ben and his mother guided me as to their needs. Ben insisted on his mother participating in every one of the five sessions that took place over two months. On reflection, this proved to be very astute of Ben, as they both engaged fully in the sessions and appeared to benefit from the process. There was a follow-up contact three months later.

In the first session we identified that the current situation felt intolerable for both of them; neither had been able to process the emotional pain of their loss (unlike Matthew); both had a similar temperament, with a need to be loved and both had taken Mr Bentley's suicide personally. Mrs Bentley also blamed herself for not seeing how depressed Mr Bentley had been.

At Ben's request, we explored in depth the idea of depression as a major illness, which can pervade a person's thoughts to the extent that it can kill. In subsequent sessions Ben reported that this reframing of Mr Bentley's death, so that it was no longer him deliberately choosing to abandon them, had greatly reduced his feelings of anger towards his father. The focus of the remaining sessions was on making sense of what had happened, dealing with the pain and learning to live again. At the last appointment both mother and son appeared to be brighter in mood, relaxed and happy. There was no evidence of clinical depression. Both reported that the sessions had helped them with the processing of their grief and both had begun to move on emotionally. Socially, Ben was gaining in confidence with his peers, mixing more and had joined a rugby club. Ben felt that the therapy had helped him to make sense of his father's death and to be able to participate in life again. He did not want any further sessions at this stage, so we agreed to review the situation three months later. At this stage Ben continued to cope well and was discharged.

Fifteen months later when I contacted Mrs Bentley and Ben to ask if I could refer to their story in a publication, it was good to learn that Ben was doing well at home, in school and socially, and that he was now able to live with what had happened. The therapy was reported to have helped both mother and son to move forward on their life journeys.

| **Box 6.8** | • What would you have done differently in Ben's case? |
| **Exercise** | • Reflect on why that might be. |

Summary

There are core counselling skills that are used in different approaches. The therapeutic relationship is identified as the vehicle for change in the models discussed. Theory is recognized as a working model to help make sense of experience. However, by emphasizing the 'human' element there is recognition that it is how we use theory, irrespective of the theoretical framework, that is essential to the counselling process. The human element includes being able to create the mental space to hold the client(s) in mind.

References

Asay, T.P. and Lambert, M.J. (2001) The empirical case for the common factors in therapy: quantitative findings, in S.G. Gowers (ed.) *Adolescent Psychiatry in Clinical Practice*. London: Arnold.

Austen, C. (2000) Integrated eclecticism: a therapeutic synthesis, in S. Palmer and R. Woofe (eds) *Integrative and Eclectic Counselling and Psychotherapy*. London: Sage.

Bowley, J. and Bratley, M. (2005) Making space for therapeutic work with adolescents and their families, *Journal of Social Work Practice*, 19(3): 289–98.

Brazier, D. (2001) *Zen Therapy: A Buddhist Approach to Psychotherapy*. London: Robinson.

Culley, S. and Bond, T. (2004) *Integrative Counselling Skills in Action*, 2nd edn. London: Sage.

Farnfield, S. and Kaszap, M. (1998) What makes a helpful grown up? Children's views of professionals in the mental health services, *Health Informatics Journal*, 4: 3–14.

Geanellos, R. (2002) Transformative change of self: the unique focus of (adolescent) mental health nursing, *International Journal of Mental Health Nursing*, 11: 174–85.

Geldard, K. and Geldard, D. (2006) Counselling children, in C. Feltham and I. Horton (eds) *The Sage Handbook of Counselling and Psychotherapy*, 2nd edn. London: Sage.

Horton, I. (2006) Integration, in C. Feltham and I. Horton (eds) *The Sage Handbook of Counselling and Psychotherapy*, 2nd edn. London: Sage.

Hunter, M. (2001) *Psychotherapy with Young People in Care: Lost and Found*. Hove: Brunner-Routledge.

Inskipp, F. (2006) Generic skills, in C. Feltham and I. Horton (eds) *The Sage Handbook of Counselling and Psychotherapy*, 2nd edn. London: Sage.

Jacobs (2004) *Psychodynamic Counselling in Action*, 3rd edn. London: Sage.

Koehn, C.V. and Cutcliffe, J.R. (2007) Hope and interpersonal psychiatric/mental health nursing: a systematic review of the literature – part one, *Journal of Psychiatric and Mental Health Nursing*, 14: 134–40.

Mearns, D. and Thorne, B. (2007) *Person-Centred Counselling in Action*, 3rd edn. London: Sage.

Peplau, H.E. (1988) *Interpersonal Relationships in Nursing*, 2nd edn. London: Macmillan.

Rogers, C.R. (1951) *Client Centred Therapy*. London: Constable.

Rogers, C.R. (1967) *On Becoming a Person*. London: Constable.

Rowan, J. and Jacobs, M. (2008) *The Therapist's Use of Self*. Maidenhead: Open University Press.

Salzberger, I. (1970) *Psycho-Analytic Insight and Relationships: A Klenian Approach*. London: Routledge.

Urwin, C. (2003) Breaking ground, hitting ground: a Sure Start rapid response service for parents and their under fours, *Journal of Child Psychotherapy*, 29(3): 375–92.

Urwin, C. (2007) Revisiting 'What works for whom?': a qualitative framework for evaluating clinical effectiveness in child psychotherapy, *Journal of Child Psychotherapy*, 33(2): 134–60.

Zack, S.E., Castongua, L.G. and Boswell, J.F. (2007) Youth Working Alliance: a core clinical construct in need of empirical maturity, *Harvard Review of Psychiatry*, 15: 278–88.

7 Family work and CAMHS nursing

Clay Frake

Key features	• Defining family work and its importance in caring.
	• Issues to consider when working with families.
	• Common challenges in family work and how to address them.

Introduction

In this chapter we look at working with families as a nurse in a child and adolescent mental health services (CAMHS) context. We discuss the importance of working with families and the challenges this may pose for the nurse. It is beyond the scope of this chapter to detail the theoretical basis and developments in family therapy – there are many good introductory text-books that do this (see Further reading, p. 95). It would also be inappropriate to suggest using highly specialized therapeutic interventions. Instead we discuss working with families as a nurse in a CAMHS context. Most of these ideas and techniques have a basis in family therapy theory and practice, but can be applied by a CAMHS nurse working within their competence and would be more properly defined as *family work*.

Family work or family therapy?

To clarify this distinction it may be helpful to briefly describe family therapy practice and how this is both different from, and similar to, how a CAMHS nurse may work with families. Family therapy draws upon a range of theories and treatment modalities. It is recognized as a distinct, separate and long established psychotherapy around the world. In the UK it takes at least four years to qualify as a family therapist with study to masters degree level. Family therapy practice is driven by the principles of collaborative working, respect for patients, recognition of the value of each individual's experience, background and beliefs and the importance of reflective practice. These are not unique to family therapy and closely match the standards outlined in the Nursing and Midwifery Council (NMC) code of practice (NMC 2008).

Family therapy sessions should be informed by a theoretical model and delivered or closely supervised by a clinician trained in that modality. *Family work* is the application of existing knowledge and experience adapted to a family context. This will often be work to complement or augment another intervention or process in the treatment. This is not intended to devalue in any way the importance of any family intervention that is delivered by a non-specialist as the success of any package of care in CAMHS will often hinge on the quality of the family work.

Why is family work so important in CAMHS work?

Working with families is a core skill for any CAMHS nurse and is one of the main differences to other areas of mental health nursing, one that many nurses find quite daunting. The family context is central to any understanding of a young person's world and any difficulties they may be experiencing. Using a risk and resilience model it becomes clear that there is huge potential for a family to influence a young person's mental health. Being comfortable and skilled at working with families is therefore central to a CAMHS nurse's effectiveness. In this chapter the focus will be on relatively formal interviews or meetings with families but will also consider some of the wider aspects of involving families in the care of a young person.

Box 7.1 The importance of family work for CAMHS nurses

- Young people are reliant on their families.
- Young people are often brought to services because of concerns about them.
- Families can help with the support and treatment for the child.

Young people in relation to families

Starting with a practical point, young people are usually reliant on their families to facilitate attendance, and their involvement in the process from the beginning is important if the young person is to access any treatment especially in an outpatient setting. A series of missed appointments in an adult service may indicate a patient's lack of engagement in the process, but this may not necessarily be the case in CAMHS. Rather, it could be a reflection of the quality of the family's engagement in the process, the working relationship between the CAMHS nurse and the family, or it may indicate practical difficulties for the family.

Children and young people do not often seek help in their own right and it is usually a parent, carer or another agency that brings any difficulties to the attention of CAMHS. This often raises issues about who is 'the customer'. Who is worried? Who is willing to make changes or help tackle the difficulty? For every member of the family there will be a different perspective and probably a different agenda. Being able to make sense of these various viewpoints and give them appropriate weighting is what makes family work so challenging and interesting.

The family's role in supporting assessment and treatment

Assessment

The family's involvement at the assessment stage is crucial. The nature of this will clearly vary depending on the developmental stage of the young person. A detailed developmental history is often needed and this is usually best provided by parents and/or carers. Young children often have very limited ways of describing their experiences and feelings so a carer's perspective is needed to formulate a clear understanding of the nature and extent of the young person's difficulties. Adolescents are usually able to give a coherent account of their difficulties but this might be from a markedly different perspective to their carers, so meeting with other members of the family will broaden the picture and enhance the quality of the assessment.

Families play a key role as partners in the care of young people. In the case of young children, parents need to give consent for an assessment and any treatment to take place. As the young person becomes competent to give their own consent (Dogra *et al.* 2009) this becomes unnecessary from a legal point of view but any package of care will be compromised if the young person's family are ambivalent or unaware of the plan. Young people presenting to CAMHS will often be facing complex, unfamiliar and frightening feelings and circumstances. The support of their families is therefore a vital component of a successful intervention. While this could equally be said of adult patients, for developmental reasons the CAMHS patient will usually have a more limited range of coping strategies and will need the support of their families as in other areas of their life.

Care planning

It is good practice to involve the family in the design of any care plan and specific intervention (being mindful, of course, of issues of confidentiality and the young person's wishes, which are discussed later in the chapter), as this brings in important elements of partnership, transparency and accountability. It also gives a clear message to the young person that everybody is working to the same end which can be reassuring and containing at a time of confusion and distress.

Ongoing support

Families often need to act as advocates for the young person in contact with CAMHS. It may be that the young person is uncertain about aspects of the care but feels unable to say so or ask for a fuller explanation, and families are often best placed to represent a young person's views. There may be serious concerns about the quality of the care and it would be an intimidating task for most young people to question this or make a formal complaint without their family's support. It can be difficult however, for the nurse faced with a question or complaint about the nature or quality of care not to experience this as an unreasonable criticism of their service or their personal qualities. It is important to remember that the role of advocate is central to that of carer and could even be described as a duty. Parents generally try to act in their children's best interests. Understanding the concerns of families and dealing with them in a straightforward and constructive way will positively influence the development of a collaborative approach to the young person's care.

Evidence base for family work

In his report on the evidence base for family interventions (Stratton 2005), commissioned by the Association of Family Therapy, Professor Stratton identified two large reviews of the evidence on the efficacy of family interventions in CAMH (Carr 2000; Cottrell and Boston 2002) which concluded that there was good evidence that these could be effective interventions in the following conditions:

- depression;
- eating disorders;
- anxiety;
- bereavement disorders;
- conduct problems;
- substance misuse;
- chronic illness;
- psycho-somatic disorders.

In addition to these extensive reviews, family interventions are recommended in the UK in the National Institute for Health and Clinical Excellence (NICE) guidelines for:

- eating disorders (NICE 2004);
- severe and moderate depression as a first-line treatment (NICE 2005).

Although some of the studies reviewed refer to specific family therapy interventions, many more, including the NICE guidelines, use a looser definition of family work and the ways of working described in this chapter match these guidelines.

Issues to consider when working with families

> **Box 7.2 Issues to consider when working with families**
>   - Who should be included?
>   - Confidentiality.
>   - What are the goals of family work (e.g. is it to support other interventions or an intervention in itself)?
>   - Setting up the meeting.
>   - Engagement.

Who should be included?

Working with a family, whether to conduct an assessment, a review or with a specific therapeutic intent, usually involves a decision about who to invite. Often the family will make this decision themselves at the first session unless specifically asked to do otherwise. Subsequent attendance will usually involve some negotiation between the family and the nurse. This naturally leads to questions about who is part of the family and who it would be appropriate to invite.

Although described as 'family' work, any work would not necessarily be limited to the immediate family. It would in any case be difficult to make a definitive description of who qualifies as a family member. This will vary with each family and perhaps each individual within that family. Families to a large extent define themselves. There will be various influences on this definition including cultural background, family disputes and the current social discourses on family. A pragmatic definition (Dogra *et al.* 2009) of family in this context would be to include everybody who is involved in meeting the child's immediate emotional and developmental needs. This could include parents and their partners, siblings, grandparents and close friends. It is important to be guided by the family's definition so as not to impose your own values on the work. Equally, it is important to be able to use your judgement regarding the presence of any individual in a meeting or involving them directly in the young person's care. The guide for this must be what you judge to be in the young person's best interests. You should be prepared however, to justify that decision with a sound rationale.

You will also need to consider the wishes of the young person, who may have strong views about who they want to be involved in their care. These views may be driven by a desire for privacy, concerns about stigma and ridicule or even fear of significant harm to themselves or others.

When undertaking any family work it is not vital that everybody in the family attends. This may be for practical reasons – a parent being unable to get time off work, for example. Families may feel that a sibling is too young to contribute to a session. Other reasons may include a discomfort with a health or therapeutic setting or even an antipathy towards the work or the young person. It may be that you decide that it would be helpful to have some sessions with different parts of the family for reasons of confidentiality or to manage a conflictual situation (see below).

Confidentiality

There are no hard and fast rules, therefore, about who should attend which sessions for family work, and while the nurse is encouraged to take a flexible approach this does however raise the issue of confidentiality. Even when restricted to members of the immediate household, practitioners may need to be mindful of this unless every member of the household has been involved in every session. If you have found it appropriate to see different parts of the family at different times there needs to be some discussion at each stage about what can be shared with whom. There may be compelling reasons why one member of the family would choose to keep some information from another, but it is important to avoid creating a complex situation with a number of secrets being kept from different members of the family. The nurse needs to give clear, unambiguous undertakings about what information will be shared. It is usually helpful to gently explore the reasons why information cannot be shared, either to get a fuller understanding of the situation or facilitate a more open discussion in the family.

At the start of a family meeting it is good practice to make a brief statement about confidentiality from your agency's perspective and develop an understanding with the family about the boundaries of any information-sharing. This is especially pertinent when working with a wider part of the family system which may include friends or other workers.

It can sometimes be difficult for parents not to be able to have access to all information about a young person's interview, but they are usually able to accept this and recognize it could be in their child's best interests if a clear explanation is given by the nurse.

Safeguarding concerns ultimately override the confidentiality of the family and if there are serious concerns about any young person's safety or well-being these have to be reported following your local protocols, even if the family have not agreed. This does not usually have to be an adversarial or secretive process and families can be involved in a collaborative way, thus preserving your working relationship.

Goals

At the beginning of the chapter we discussed the difference between family therapy and family work and it is important to be clear about that distinction when looking at what the CAMHS nurse might hope to achieve when working with families. While there are many occasions where a family-based intervention will be the sole or main treatment modality in CAMHS, these would usually come into the realm of family therapy and require a separate set of skills. Here we look at the realistic goals of what might be achieved by the CAMHS nurse.

Box 7.3 Exercise	You have been asked to complete a risk assessment on a 13-year-old girl who has been admitted to the accident & emergency (A&E) ward following an overdose of analgesics. Her parents are available but she does not want you to meet with them. Her father is angry and demanding to talk to you. • What dilemmas does this present you with? • What would you do next?

Reviewing progress for individual work

The need to involve families in the assessment process is clear but it is equally important for them to be involved at regular reviews of any ongoing work with a young person. This is particularly important if the intervention is largely individual work. Reviews can be used to check if the care plan is still relevant, address any difficulties that might be emerging in the work, provide another perspective to check on progress, and at the end of any work.

Psycho-education

The role of psycho-education with the family is especially important in CAMHS work. Depending on their developmental stage, the young person may not have a full understanding of the process and may need other members of the family to help them with this alongside the nurse. Families will usually want to know more about a diagnosis or treatment. It is important to remember that in a similar way to the young person coming into contact with CAMHS for the first time, members of the family may be feeling bewildered and distressed about the situation. Parents and siblings often blame themselves for any difficulties and this can be usefully explored with the family. By developing an understanding of a condition or set of difficulties the family are better placed to help. This can be particularly useful for siblings, who can feel disempowered and distanced from their brother's or sister's experiences. There will often be different perceptions and beliefs about the mental health needs of the young person within the family or wider system and this can lead to an unintentional undermining of any intervention. The nurse needs to give a clear rationale for any intervention and answer the family's questions openly and to the best of their knowledge. It may also be helpful to discuss the different views and beliefs of the family and, if appropriate, explore the basis of these ideas. An intervention is much more likely to succeed if it takes this into account.

Box 7.4 Case scenario

Gemma is a 16-year-old girl who has a moderate to severe depression which has failed to respond to psychological therapies. A psychiatrist colleague has prescribed antidepressant medication and Gemma is willing to try this as she wants to feel better. Gemma's mother is in agreement but her father is unhappy about the idea. He is angry with the team for suggesting this and says he will stop her coming to any more sessions. A meeting with parents only is arranged and when this ambivalence is discussed in more detail it emerges that several members of his family had been treated with medication for mental health problems in the past and he found the thought of Gemma doing the same deeply upsetting. By talking about this openly and thinking about Gemma's individual needs he was able to let her make her own decision about medication and was also able to be much more involved in her treatment and recovery.

Family work as an adjunct to other interventions

Family work alongside other interventions is often used to great effect in CAMHS work. It has the potential to enlist other family members in a collaborative approach to any care and generate creative ways of working. Many mental health problems can be frightening for a young person to tackle on their own and the support or direct involvement of their family can be very reassuring. Any improvements are much more likely to be generalized and sustained if more people are aware of the efforts made by the young person or are making a contribution to the therapeutic work. If individual work has reached an impasse or there are problems with compliance, working with the family can be a useful forum to explore possible reasons for the loss of impetus and to re-energize the process. The benefits of including the family to enhance any work will, of course, need to be balanced against issues of confidentiality and the young person's wishes.

Issues to consider when family work is an adjunct to other interventions

There are some important issues to consider when working with a family in parallel to other interventions. Firstly, should the family work involve the same person who is offering the other intervention? For reasons of economy or convenience this is often the case and the advisability of this depends to a great extent on the nature of the work being undertaken. If, for example, the work was a relatively straightforward intervention to address a specific phobia then it would seem appropriate for the nurse doing this work to meet regularly with the family to review the progress and involve them with any homework. If the work was of a different nature such regular individual sessions looking at intensely personal feelings and developing alternative coping strategies, then it may be much less helpful for the nurse to be seeing both the young person and other members of the family. The young person can often come to regard the nurse in this situation as 'their' worker and might be resentful of sharing them with their parents or fearful of breaches in confidentiality. If the decision is taken to allocate the work to different clinicians then particular care needs to be taken over communication and it is helpful to have frequent discussions to maintain a coherence to the work and prevent differences emerging in the two strands, which can develop into splitting, where two clinicians identify with competing and often conflictual perspectives. In practice it is usually feasible for the nurse to see both the young person and their family even in relatively complex cases, providing care is taken over developmentally appropriate negotiation between the young person and the nurse about boundaries regarding information-sharing. This also puts the nurse in a good position to act as advocate for the young person if necessary. Other variations on this can work well, especially in highly complex cases, with the nurse doing the individual work accompanying the young person to family meetings or reviews conducted by a colleague. If necessary the nurse can help the young person prepare for the session, support them in discussing any difficult issues and reflect on the session afterwards.

CBT is often used as an evidenced-based approach to a range of problems in young people and is an exemplar of how individual work can be usefully enhanced by working with the family. Families can help elaborate on a young person's understanding of their difficulties and any intervention can work alongside the young person to complete homework tasks or encourage them apply suggested strategies. However, you should bear in mind that the impact of at least some members of the family has the potential to be much greater than even weekly sessions with a clinician. Sometimes the instinctive responses of families in search of solutions have unwittingly become part of the problem.

Box 7.5 Case scenario

Smita is an 11-year-old girl who was referred to CAMHS with a generalized anxiety; she became distressed when her parents left the house in case they had an accident, she frequently asked for reassurance about her own health and needed her mother to lie next to her in bed before she could go to sleep. Both parents had become caught up in a cycle of reassurance with their anxious child. Their attempts to assuage specific fears began to generate higher levels of anxiety in an escalating process. The attempted CBT intervention was making little headway as Smita's parents found it hard to allow her to experience any distress. They found the responses recommended by the nurse to Smita's need for reassurance to be counter-intuitive and couldn't always follow the advice.

Smita's mother disclosed that she also had been very anxious as a child and although this no longer affected her functioning, she could easily identify with Smita. The family work helped the parents develop a good understanding of the condition and intervention, and Smita's mother's own experience of anxiety was used as a resource rather than a hindrance as she had overcome her own childhood difficulty in this respect.

When it might not be appropriate to meet with the family as a single unit

It may be that in any stage of the work there are compelling developmental reasons why it may not be appropriate to work with the family all together, at least initially. These might include discussion of difficulties in a parental relationship which are impacting on a young person's mental health, or an adolescent discussing issues about their sexuality. A frequent reason for working with families together with individual work is the sense that the differences within the family may be too wide to work with initially. This gap may exist for a wide range of reasons but the goal here will be to gradually bring the two parallel strands together. The practicalities of this are discussed later in the chapter.

Working with the family

Engagement

The beginning and initial phase of any family work needs careful thought and preparation. It sets the scene for future work and influences the family's attendance at any subsequent sessions. It is usually complicated by having to take several people's needs and perspectives into consideration.

Preparation

The preparation starts with the method of invitation to the family work. This is usually by letter but can be arranged in another venue or over the telephone. The invitation is usually addressed to the main carers of the family as they will have to facilitate any attendance. This initial contact should include a clear explanation of what to expect and a brief explanation of the rationale for working with the family. It is probably best not to go into too much detail at this point as any questions can be explored more thoroughly at the meeting and with everyone who attends.

Gaining the family's confidence

At the outset the nurse needs to project an air of confidence and familiarity with the process to contain any anxieties or ambivalence the family might be experiencing. It is important to remember that in this context the nurse is on familiar territory and is probably meeting with families regularly, whereas the family may be facing an entirely new experience. Equally, as the aim is to work collaboratively with the family, it is essential that they retain a sense of being expert on their own predicament. If necessary, some ground rules can be negotiated about respectful ways of communicating in the session. It can be useful to remind members of the family that they have the option of being seen separately if necessary if there are concerns about the appropriateness of sharing information.

Introductions and explanations

Starting with introductions is an obvious point but this can be a good opportunity to enhance the engagement. One technique is to ask one of the younger members of the family or the referred young person to introduce their family. It is vital to play close attention to the names and style of address – for instance, that paternal grandmother is called 'Nana', as this helps prevent a family feel they are 'just another case'. A good opening question is to ask everybody at the meeting – including the nurse – to describe their understanding of why they have been asked to meet. If each individual is given a chance to speak this can be quite a long process, but it serves to clarify expectations and models a respectful style of talking in the session. Goal-setting discussions with the family should be central to the engagement process as this gives a relevance and direction to the family work. As with all goals these should be realistic, measurable and meaningful for all concerned, with a timescale for review. Where this differs in family work is the likelihood that this will involve some negotiation.

Summarizing the process

Finally, it can be helpful to end the initial session with a brief reflection on the process so far; has it met their expectations? Would they like a further session? What do they think it will be useful to address next time? Has anything been said that needs further clarification?

Box 7.6 Common challenges in family work

- Moving away from blaming the family or an individual.
- Managing arguments or conflict in the session.
- Engaging reluctant participants.

Common challenges in family work

Moving away from blaming the family

Contact with a CAMHS, especially first contact, can be a very stressful time for families. It is a natural response of a parent when faced with a child's mental health problem to question their own role in the creation of the problem. In the past, various therapeutic models have blamed parents, particularly mothers, for causing a range of psychiatric and developmental problems. Although these views have largely been rejected by modern evidence-based practice they still carry some weight in popular culture and consequently affect parents and families. This is not to imply that parents' behaviour is not a significant contributing factor in the mental health problems of many young people or to absolve adults of responsibility for their actions, but to caution against institutional assumptions. The very act of asking the family to be part of any intervention is often interpreted as an implication that they are in some way to blame.

Any family or parent who is feeling blamed is likely to enter into family work in fairly guarded way. This effect can be magnified if the parent has experienced a similar condition to their child. A good starting point is to ask the family what they thought about being asked to join the work and explore any themes that emerge. It can be helpful to emphasize that the family can play a central role in the young person's recovery and that they are regarded as part of the solution rather than part of the problem. Conversely, if it emerges that the parents have a strong self-imposed sense that they are in some way to blame for their child's difficulties, it is important not to dismiss this out of hand but spend some time discussing how they came to this belief and how it might be affecting their actions. It is usually more constructive to take a pragmatic approach to blame: is it more or less likely to help the young person with whom you are working?

Moving away from blaming the child

The usual procedure of asking about the young person's difficulties naturally invites discussion about the more negative aspects of their behaviour. This often happens when parents feel threatened or that they have not been listened to by other agencies. If this discussion becomes prolonged or particularly critical it can be distressing for the young person and uncomfortable for the clinician. It is important however to allow the parents some opportunity to speak about their worries and frustrations if they are to feel that their concerns are being taken seriously. If the meeting becomes stuck at this point there are several strategies which may be helpful to interrupt the process. The young person can be brought into the conversation by either directly asking for their views or by inviting the parents to take their child's perspective. The conversation can be moved in a more positive direction by asking about attempted solutions to the problem and the parents' hopes for any intervention. This has the added effect of placing the parents back in the role as experts on their own children.

Despite attempts to manage the situation, the session may become too difficult, even to the point where the nurse feels they are in danger of colluding with an abusive exchange and it would be more appropriate to meet separately with different parts of the family, at least initially.

Arguments in family meetings

A young person's referral to CAMHS often puts a family under a lot of stress and in these circumstances it is not surprising that conflicts within the family are often played out in family meetings, even in subtle ways. This may be between parent and child, siblings, partners and ex-partners. Because the nurse's role is often perceived as a professional expert, they may be invited to take sides and confirm one party's perspective. Observing such conflicts can give useful insights into the context of a young person's difficulties and these are usually issues about which strong feelings are held, but discussion can quickly deteriorate into a shouting match. The nurse, who has probably asked the family to attend in the first place, may feel a tremendous pressure to rescue the meeting from chaos. At this point their role may be more likened to a referee rather than a mediator. The temptation may be to quickly arrive at a consensus or to promote one particular view, but this approach is probably doomed to fail especially if it is early in the process. The task is to manage the session rather than try to make the differences 'go away'. The nurse may have to take firm control of the session and should feel able to interrupt an individual if the discussion becomes destructive. This can be done in a respectful way, for example, 'I'm sorry to interrupt but I wanted to hear what your son thinks about this.' It is important to use a form of words which feel comfortable but it is surprising how a direction will be complied with if made respectfully and firmly but with a smile. Focusing on the process rather than the content of an argument can take some of the heat out of an exchange and shift perspectives. Examples of this might be, 'How do arguments usually start at home and how are they resolved?' or 'When your dad and sister argue, what do you do?' This moves the conversation away from the need to score points and gives the participants a brief opportunity to reflect on a pattern of interaction.

Reluctant participants

Young people often find it hard to talk in meetings. This can be for a variety of reasons including embarrassment, anxiety, anger and fear of ridicule, or even repercussions after the meeting; or it may be that they cannot find the words to express themselves. While it may not be immediately apparent why they are not speaking, it is important to give them the opportunity to participate. It can be useful to state that just as they have a right to have their voice heard it is also fine for them to say nothing. This usually takes the pressure off the young person and at the very least allows them to listen to what others are saying without being preoccupied with the fear that someone is going to make them speak. By periodically returning to them to check their views, they can choose to review their wish to speak without any loss of face. Sometimes the technique of offering multiple choice answers can help the most reticent young people contribute to the session. A range of responses can be offered to which the young person can simply nod or shake their head. Rating scales can often be used to good effect when a young person is struggling to articulate their feelings. If the young person is gently included without being pushed to speak they will often find their voice later in the session or at subsequent meetings.

Sometimes, members of the family do not attend meetings for practical reasons or as a result of an unwillingness to participate at that point. It is important to keep open the possibility that they might attend in the future by keeping them engaged, albeit in a peripheral way, with the family work. The simplest way to do this is to ask the family who will be able to update any absent members on what is happening in the family work. This can be revisited at future sessions as a way of keeping all of the family in mind.

Record-keeping

As with all note-taking, it is important that the record of the session is contemporaneous and concise, and a clear distinction made between fact and speculation. Where key phrases are recorded these should be placed in quotation marks. Recording of family sessions differs from individual sessions in the number of participants and the interactions between them. A useful way to organize this is to separately record the *themes* of the session (e.g. the main areas of discussion) and the *process* – qualitative information such as how the discussion was conducted, who talked the most/least, the non-verbal communication and so on.

Summary

This chapter has summarized how the main techniques from family therapy can be applied in everyday nursing practice in working with families. It is important to be aware of the distinction between family work and family therapy, as the latter is a very specific way of working and requires specialist training. The skills to undertake family work are important for nurses to acquire and practise in delivering CAMHS.

References

Carr (2000) Evidence-based practice in family therapy and systemic consultation I: child focused problems, *Journal of Family Therapy*, 22: 29–60.

Cottrell, D. and Boston, P. (2002) Practitioner review: the effectiveness of systemic family therapy for children and adolescents, *Journal of Child Psychology and Psychiatry*, 43(5): 573–86.

Dogra, N., Parkin, A., Gale, F. and Frake, C. (2009) *A Multidisciplinary Handbook of Child and Adolescent Mental Health for Front-line Professionals*. London: Jessica Kingsley.

NICE (National Institute for Health and Clinical Excellence) (2004) *Clinical Guidelines for Eating Disorders*. London: NICE.

NICE (National Institute for Health and Clinical Excellence) (2005) *Clinical Guidelines for Depression in Children and Young People*. London: NICE.

NMC (Nursing and Midwifery Council) (2008) *The Code: Standards of Conduct, Performance and Ethics for Nurses and Midwives*, www.nmc-uk.org/AArticle.aspx?ArticleID=3057, accessed 20 August 2008.

Stratton P. (2005) *Report on the Evidence Base of Systemic Family Therapy*. Warrington: Association for Family Therapy.

Further reading

Burnham, J.B. (1986) *Family Therapy*. London: Tavistock Library of Social Work Practice.

Carr, A. (2000) *Family Therapy: Concepts, Process and Practice*. Chichester: Wiley.

Wilson, J. (1998) *Child-focused Practice: A Collaborative Systemic Approach*. London: Karnac.

8 | Cognitive behavioural therapy and the CAMH nurse

Michael Hodgkinson

Key features	• The theoretical origins of cognitive behavioural therapy (CBT).
	• The evidence base for use of CBT with different child and adolescent mental health problems.
	• CBT formulations as a means of understanding and presenting problems.
	• CBT approaches as a means of effective intervention.

Introduction

In this chapter, we will look at how the principles of CBT can be applied to inform a child and adolescent mental health (CAMH) nurse's work with children, young people and families. As with other types of therapy, it requires specialist training to work formally as a cognitive behavioural therapist and this chapter does not aim to equip the CAMH nurse to practise at that level. Rather, it will cover the theoretical background to CBT; the evidence base for its use with children and young people; the way in which CBT formulations can be used to help the practitioner *understand* what is causing or maintaining problems; and how CBT approaches can then be used to *address* those problems. Finally, for those who may wish to read further, some more specialized texts are referenced at the end of the chapter.

The theoretical basis of CBT

Animal learning theories – classical and operant conditioning

In the first part of the twentieth century, experiments were undertaken to discover the mechanisms by which animals learn. It is not possible to cover this work in detail here, but one of the main names associated with these developments is Pavlov, a Russian physiologist who identified the mechanisms of 'classical conditioning' in his famous experiments with dogs. Some years later on the other side of the Atlantic, Skinner conducted a series of studies with pigeons and rats, and identified the rules of 'operant learning'.

Classical conditioning

Pavlov (1927), investigating the salivary reflex in dogs, observed that under certain conditions they could be trained to salivate in response to non-food cues. He used the terms 'stimulus' and 'response' to denote the trigger and the behaviour resulting from it, respectively.

In his experiments, food was the *unconditioned stimulus* (UCS), as it would naturally produce salivation, which was termed the *unconditioned response* (UCR). By ringing a bell at the same time as presenting the food, over a series of trials the bell gradually became a *conditioned stimulus* (CS) – because it would only activate the salivary response *on condition* that it was presented at the same time as food (see Figure 8.1). Once this learning was established, the sound of the bell alone would produce salivation (as a conditioned response – CR). How often has your stomach rumbled in anticipation when you have looked at your watch and noticed it's lunchtime? That is classical conditioning at work.

Pavlov also noted that:

- the CS and UCS need to be closely connected in time to produce a CR;
- if a CS stops predicting the appearance of the UCS, its power gradually extinguishes;
- *generalization* occurs as stimuli similar to the CS may also produce the CR.

Operant conditioning

Classical conditioning could explain the acquisition and maintenance of some behaviours. However, in order to account for the development of new pieces of voluntary behaviour, the notion of *operant conditioning* was required. Thorndike (1911), from observations of animal learning, suggested that behaviours that secured a positive consequence would be more likely to be repeated in the future than those that did not – the *law of effect*. Skinner (1938) introduced a new term into the law of effect – *reinforcement*. Simply stated, behaviour that is *reinforced* tends to be strengthened: behaviour which is not reinforced tends to die out – or *extinguish*.

Skinner's experiments studied operant conditioning in rats and pigeons through use of the 'Skinner box'. These contained a bar to press or a disk to peck and food was delivered to the animal dependent upon them performing a specific behaviour. Initially the animal's exploration of the box would result in them 'accidentally' performing the required action, which would result in the delivery of the food. No other actions would be rewarded. Under these conditions, learning takes place relatively quickly – and is even more accelerated through the process of *shaping* or *successive approximation*. In classical conditioning the UCS itself provides the reinforcement. In operant conditioning, the reinforcement is presented *after* the response. These points are illustrated in Figures 8.2 to 8.5.

Negative reinforcement involves *removing a negative response* (such as low-level electric shock in Skinner's experiments) to reinforce the occurrence of a target behaviour.

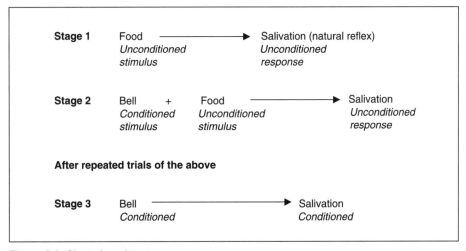

Figure 8.1 Classical conditioning

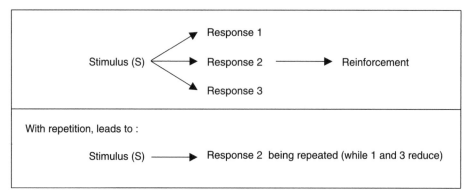

Figure 8.2 Positive reinforcement

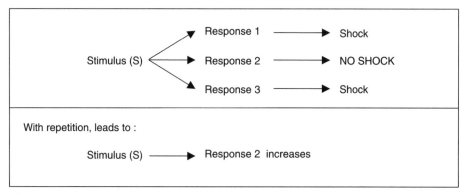

Figure 8.3 Negative reinforcement: this involves *removing a negative response* (such as low-level electric shock in Skinner's experiments) to reinforce the occurrence of a target behaviour

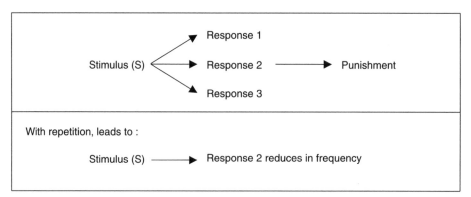

Figure 8.4 Punishment

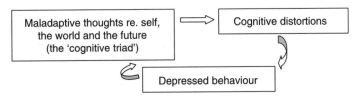

Figure 8.5 The relationship between cognitive distortion and mood

Key points about operant conditioning

- For learning to occur, the response has to follow quickly after the stimulus (so, for instance, punishing a child's behaviour hours after it has occurred does not allow learning to occur).
- The relationship between the stimulus and the response needs to be consistent over a number of trials in order for learning to occur (so praising a child very occasionally for behaving well is unlikely to produce an overall increase in positive behaviour).
- 'Shaping' refers to an operant process by which behaviour can be changed towards a desired end target through a series of gradual steps (such as when teaching a toddler to spoon feed and gradually increasing in accuracy!).

Applying animal learning to human behaviour

Once these theories of animal learning had been established, the question of their applicability to human behaviour was raised. Would the same principles of classical and operant conditioning hold for a dog, a pigeon and a person? Although we may not be too happy to hear it, there is strong evidence that the principles governing the way pigeons and rats behave also apply to us. However, the hallmark of any learning that occurs as a result of classical or operant conditioning is that the animal (or person) has to *directly experience* the relationship between the stimulus and the response. This cannot account for all human behaviour and attitudes. For example, most of us learn that murder is wrong without having to murder someone and suffer the consequences. What other type of learning is responsible for this, and how does it work?

Social learning theory

The essence of both classical and operant conditioning is that the organism's behaviour is moulded through *directly experiencing* associations between stimuli and response. However, in the 1970s, social learning theorists such as Mischel (1976) and Bandura (1977) developed the idea that the *expectations* of reward and punishment and *observation* of the outcome of other individuals' behaviour might also play an important role in the acquisition of social and more complex behaviours.

The role of *imitation* is central to these theories and they propose that through *vicarious reinforcement* (observing the outcomes of other people's behaviour), patterns of behaviour may be developed or avoided without the individual having to directly experience their consequences.

Social learning has been suggested as an explanation for the acquisition of complex behaviours such as morality, sex roles and attitudes; and conversely, for the development of aggressive and antisocial behaviours. It can also provide a means of understanding the cause of clinically-presenting problem behaviours and define the targets for intervention.

The addition of social learning theory enabled us to account for a much wider range of human behaviours than classical and operant conditioning alone. The combination of the three provided a framework for us to understand how some unwanted behaviours (such as phobias and aggressive or antisocial behaviours) may have come about – and also how we could intervene to effect positive change. The application of learning theory to help change human behaviour has been known variously over the years as 'behaviour modification', and more latterly as 'behaviour therapy'. It is important to note that this is not only a means of reducing problematic behaviours (either a problem for the individual or for those around him/her), but also an effective way of building on positives to help individuals acquire or enhance new skills.

From behaviour therapy to CBT

Although the focus on observable and quantifiable behaviours was seen by many as a welcome development, others found the exclusive emphasis on external behaviours too *reductionist*. Such critics proposed that human beings do not simply generate behaviours through stimulus-response relationships, but we also have thoughts, emotions, memories and motivations that influence the way in which we understand or make sense of the world. It is not only what happens that influences our behaviour, but more what we *believe* has happened and the sense we make of it. Shakespeare's Hamlet put it like this: 'There's nothing either good or bad, but thinking makes it so'.

This suggests that the relationship between stimulus and response is not simple and unchangeable, but that it is strongly mediated by the way we think about and understand it. The addition of recognizing the role of cognitions (thoughts) in influencing behaviour brought about the move from behaviour therapy to CBT.

Early CBT models

Rational emotive therapy

Albert Ellis (1957) identified the link between behaviour, emotions and cognitions in his rational emotive therapy (RET). The essence of this was that emotions and resulting behaviours depend on how events are cognitively construed, rather than springing from the event per se.

Ellis proposed that when any event occurs (which he called 'activating events'), we spontaneously generate a variety of beliefs to try to make sense of what has happened. According to which of the possible beliefs we decide to accept, there will be different emotional consequences for us (hence, we have the activating event, leading to beliefs, leading in turn to emotional consequences). Ellis also stressed that beliefs may be *rational* or *irrational*, and that acceptance of irrational beliefs is more likely in individuals who are depressed, anxious or with low self-esteem. Not only are such individuals more likely to adopt such beliefs, but the emotional consequences of doing so form a vicious cycle, perpetuating their negative mood states.

Box 8.1 Exercise	• Imagine walking into a room, and as you do so, a group already there burst into laughter (activating event). What beliefs would you have to account for that event? Are they laughing at you? Did you walk in at the punchline of a joke – a coincidence? Are they a happy group who laugh all the time anyway?

- If, having weighed up the possibilities, you conclude that Belief 1 is correct (they were laughing specifically at you), how would that make you feel? If, however, you decided that one of the other beliefs was more likely to be correct (i.e it is nothing personal about you), would the event have the same effect on you?
- Finally, what if your current mental state (depressed, highly anxious, low self-esteem) is distorting your idea of what is rational and irrational (which we know it will)? What emotional consequences is that likely to have? How could we change that?

Helping the individual first to recognize, and then to challenge irrational beliefs is the basis of the therapeutic approach in RET.

Cognitive therapy

Aaron Beck (1970) is generally credited as another of the first to link a variety of psychological problems (such as depression) to maladaptive or 'distorted' cognitions (1970) as shown in Figure 8.5. He was also the first to adopt the term 'cognitive therapy' in the literature, although this has since come to be used as an umbrella term for a range of therapies in which attention to cognitive processes forms the main focus.

Beck's model included the notion of *core beliefs* or *schemas*, which he defined as relatively fixed beliefs, often determined by early experience, and against which current events are assessed. These fixed beliefs, when activated by an event, produce negative automatic thoughts (NATs), which in turn lead to cognitive distortions and thereafter depressed mood. Figure 8.6 shows the linkages between the different parts of the model. It also highlights that such cognitive distortions have emotional, behavioural and somatic consequences for the individual.

Beck's work asserted that distorted cognitions may induce negative emotional states. This model was further developed by John Teasdale (Teasdale and Fogarty 1979), whose experiments

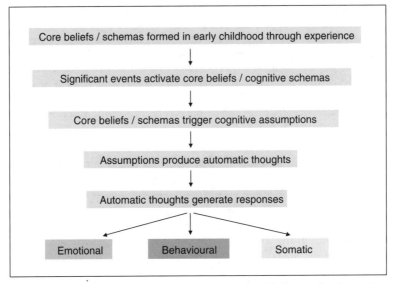

Figure 8.6 The different components that link emotional, behavioural and somatic responses

on 'induced moods' established evidence for a two-way relationship between emotional states and cognitions. Not only do distorted cognitions lead to negative emotional states (as Beck found), but negative feelings can also produce distorted cognitions. They are therefore *interdependent*.

The evidence base for CBT in CAMHS

There is a broad and increasing evidence base for the use of CBT with children and young people presenting with a variety of problems. These include:

- generalized anxiety disorders (e.g. Kendall 1994);
- fears and phobias (e.g. King *et al.* 2005);
- depressive disorders (e.g. Harrington *et al.* 1998);
- social phobia (Spence *et al.* 2000);
- school refusal (King *et al.* 1998);
- conduct problems (Herbert 1978);
- obsessive-compulsive disorder (OCD) (March 2005).

In addition, CBT approaches are being recommended as the first-line treatment in a succession of condition-specific guidelines from the National Institute for Health and Clinical Excellence (NICE) within the CAMH field (including depression, deliberate self-harm, anorexia nervosa, specific anxiety disorders, OCD and body dysmorphic disorder, post-traumatic stress disorder – PTSD, and attention deficit hyperactivity disorder – ADHD; for more details see the NICE website, www.nice.org.uk):

At this point in time then, CBT has established itself as the form of therapy most strongly backed by scientific evidence for most, though not all, forms of child and adolescent psychiatric disorder. Other forms of therapy are, nevertheless, widely applied on the assumption that lack of evidence for their effectiveness does not constitute evidence for ineffectiveness.

(Graham 2005: 60)

It is important to note that despite evidence for its effectiveness with a variety of clinical conditions, CBT is not a panacea for all. Although there is compelling evidence for its short-term effectiveness in many areas, studies that have looked at longer-term durability of effects generally find less impressive results. However, we need to bear in mind that most of the research evidence comes from a US context and often will be from work with highly selected examples which may not reflect the complexity of everyday clinical practice. There is clearly still work to be done, but the CBT approach offers the CAMH nurse a framework within which to form an understanding of a client's presenting problems, and a set of principles to guide therapeutic interventions in CBT casework.

Applying the principles of a CBT approach to aid the nurse's understanding of 'real-life' clinical problems

One of the most helpful CBT frameworks to make sense of how certain behaviours develop and are maintained is that of *applied behavioural analysis* (ABA). This involves analysing a specific behaviour in terms of the context in which it occurs (the *antecedents*); and with regard to the result it achieves for the individual (the *consequences*).

Antecedents describes the context in which the behaviour occurs. They may be environmental factors (such as time of day, place, other individuals who are present etc.) or internal states (such as mood, level of anxiety or stress, boredom etc.).

The behaviour must be defined in clear, operational terms (avoid vague or general terms like 'naughty', 'aggressive', 'rude', since these may mean different things to different people).

The *consequences* are the result of the behaviour. It is vital that we look at how the child or young person experiences the result – not how we as adults might perceive it. So how do we put antecedents, behaviour and consequences together to make sense of a specific behaviour that has been targeted for our attention? Table 8.1 gives examples of the types of information we need to gather under each heading.

Table 8.1 Putting the information together

Antecedents ⟶	Behaviour ⟶	Consequences
When?	Precisely defined	What are the *obvious results* of the behaviour?
Where?		
Who with?		
Mood state?		
Level of self-esteem		Any less obvious but equally *real* results?
Stressors		
Temperament		
ANTECEDENTS ⟶	BEHAVIOUR ⟶	CONSEQUENCE
Low self-esteem?	Sits with arms folded and refuses to work	Boy is sent out of the classroom
Numeracy difficulty?		Relieves boy of pressure to perform
Self-conscious about problem		Preserves some self-esteem through avoiding detection

Box 8.2 Case scenario

- Consider now how you might use the ABC format to make sense of the a real-life situation described below.

A 9-year-old boy refuses to work in his class at school, usually when the class is doing numeracy. The teacher warns him about his behaviour, but when the behaviour gets worse the boy is sent out of the lesson to stand in the corridor. This seems to be happening more and more.

- Why might the boy be behaving in this way? Take a few minutes to think about this before reading on.

In the case outlined in Box 8.2, the ABA model would ask the following questions:

- What are the antecedents to this behaviour?
- How can we define the behaviour in precise terms?
- What is the consequence of the behaviour for the boy?

Analysis

The analysis suggests that the 'negative' behaviour may be performing a 'positive' function for the child (in preserving some self-esteem) and is therefore being actively maintained. Note that the teacher no doubt thinks she is *punishing* the student for his non-compliance – whereas in fact his behaviour is being *rewarded* by being excluded from a task in which he expects to experience failure or social exposure. Once we understand this, it makes sense that his behaviour is not changing as we now have a 'working hypothesis' about what is driving the behaviour, and what is maintaining it. The same working hypothesis can point the clinician to where changes might be effected in order to produce the desired shift in the behaviour. In this way, the behavioural analysis can be developed into a behavioural intervention.

In this example, intervention might include:

- working on the antecedents to remove the context for the behaviour (e.g. building the child's self-esteem and providing extra academic support to the child to promote his sense of success in the lesson)
- changing the consequences so that they no longer positively reinforce the child's negative behaviour (e.g by keeping the child within the classroom for the numeracy lesson but using a different sanction).

In practice, adults tend naturally to focus more on the 'consequences' part of the process when trying to produce a behavioural change, but the most helpful and effective changes are often made at the 'antecedent' end. There is also an important ethical dimension to the issue.

In the example above, the suggested changes that might be achieved in the antecedents would not only make the non-compliant behaviour pointless and unnecessary for the child, but they would also enhance his self-esteem. Changing the sanction used for his non-compliance might well reduce that specific behaviour as it is no longer serving the function of achieving his escape from the class – *but* it would do nothing to address his self-esteem issues and might even make these worse. He would now be more confronted by his problems, without offering him any new support in managing them. Which of these seems the better outcome for the boy?

Finally, although the title of ABA might imply that it is only interested in observable behaviours, the worked example above illustrates that it can, and should, also include information about the feelings, perceptions, cognitions and even value systems associated with them. The working hypothesis generated by the ABA is tested by making changes in the antecedents and/or consequences surrounding the target behaviour. If, over time, the behaviour does not change as the hypothesis would predict, the ABA should be revisited. This makes the process particularly robust and the clinician should never be afraid to change the working hypothesis in the light of new information.

Using CBT-informed interventions

CBT is not a single entity, but rather a collection of therapeutic approaches that involve promoting change for people in their behavioural and/or cognitive processes. The focus for change may be the young person, the parent, or both, and CBT provides a range of possible approaches that can be matched to individual needs. For example, Stallard (2004) suggested that as young children are cognitively immature, they are more likely to benefit from more behaviour-based interventions, since they may lack the insight required to identify and modify their own cognitions.

At the same time, although cognitive-based approaches are generally more successful in treating anxiety disorders, the opposite is true of conduct disorders, where behaviour-based interventions are more effective. Both argue for using a range of therapeutic techniques across the cognitive-behavioural continuum, according to the type of presenting problem and level of cognitive development.

Examples of using behaviour therapy

Behaviour therapy techniques (based on learning theory principles) may be used to:

- teach new behaviours – such as dressing, personal hygiene and pro-social skills;
- address areas of behavioural *deficits* – where age-appropriate behaviours are either absent or occur at an inappropriately low frequency (in these situations the objective is to increase the frequency and/or intensity of the behaviour to a more appropriate level);
- address areas of behavioural *excesses* – behaviours that occur at an inappropriately high frequency or intensity (such as frequent or extreme anger outbursts) where the objective is to reduce the frequency and/or intensity of the behaviour to a more socially acceptable level;
- maintain existing positive behaviours.
- change maladaptive behaviours where 'faulty learning' has taken place (e.g. phobias and anxiety states where extreme fear responses have become conditioned to environmental stimuli that are not inherently threatening, such as children who are faecally incontinent because they have become fearful of opening their bowels on a toilet, and consequently avoid using it, with soiling the inevitable consequence).

Examples of using of CBT

At the other end of the CBT continuum, cognitively-based interventions are more helpful where the focus for change is around addressing cognitive distortions, rather than changing behaviour per se. For example:

- there is evidence that anxious children tend to misperceive neutral stimuli as being threatening; that they tend to be excessively self-focused and critical; and that they report negative expectations of the future (Kendall and Panichelli-Mindel 1995);
- aggressive children tend to misperceive others' neutral intent as aggressive; they have fewer cognitive problem-solving skills to manage interpersonal issues and base their assumptions of other people's intent toward them on relatively fewer cues (Dodge 1980);
- depressed children and young people are more likely to attribute negative events to internal, stable causes, which in terms of attribution theory implies that they somehow 'own' the negative events (internal) and see them as a constant feature of their lives (stable); conversely, they tend to attribute positive events to external and unstable causes (paraphrasing, 'It's nothing to do with me and it won't last anyway').

In relation to all the examples above, it is evident that the focus for change is not necessarily the child's behaviour in all cases, but rather their interpretation and cognitive understanding of what is happening around them. These cognitive distortions may indeed have behavioural consequences that need to be managed, but it is somewhat missing the point if the behaviours are responded to without addressing the distorted cognitions from which they emanate.

For example, consider the case of a young person who is referred to clinical services for 'anger management'. Some such individuals will share other people's concern about their angry outbursts and will be motivated to achieve greater control for themselves. They may well benefit from being taught self-control techniques using behavioural or cognitive strategies, or both. However, if the young person feels justified in becoming angry and aggressive with peers because he misperceives them as being hostile towards him, why would he want to control his 'righteous' anger? If this is ever going to occur, it will be after he has learned to interpret his peers' behaviour in a less hostile way, so successful intervention at a *cognitive* level is vital if the *behavioural* issues are to become accessible to change.

Application in practice

A comprehensive account of the behavioural and cognitive approaches that might be subsumed under the CBT mantle in CAMH work is beyond the scope of this chapter, but some useful 'key points' can be extracted to define the approach.

1 Engagement. The CBT approach requires *active collaboration* between therapist and client, and this is unlikely to be possible without a level of rapport and trust being achieved. Given that cognitions are internal events, the therapist is entirely dependent upon the client choosing to share these.

2 A sound assessment is a prerequisite of an informed intervention – otherwise you may be wasting the client's (and your own) time.

   a Be aware that what a parent reports about their child's behaviour is not necessarily objective 'truth', but is rather their perception of what happens. This can be influenced by various factors such as parental mental state, levels of expectation, parental belief systems and many others.

   b It is safest to base assessments on as broad an evidence base as possible, preferably obtaining information from more than one adult and from more than one setting (such as home and school). Discrepancies in what is reported may reflect that the child does indeed present very differently in combination with different adults or across settings, which is very useful information. Many children whose behaviour is very challenging and non-compliant within the home do not present in that way within the structured, less emotional environment of school. This suggests that the behavioural problems are not inevitable or inherent, but controlled by environmental context.

   c Alternatively, the inconsistencies in what is reported may be a reflection of the same behaviour being experienced as problematic by one parent, for instance, but as 'normal' by the other. One parent feels the child has a 'problem'. The other disagrees, so if the assessment is based on either informant alone, the conclusions are likely to be unhelpfully skewed one way or another.

   d Asking carers (or the child/young person if appropriate) to record the daily incidence of target behaviours on a chart over a period of time can be effective in finding out what is actually occurring. An overwhelmed and exhausted parent may well feel that their child exhibits the same problem behaviours invariably, day in and day out, whereas objective recording usually reveals that there are variations in the pattern, with some days being markedly less problematic than others. This discovery helps people to feel less hopeless about the problem and the pattern over time can produce very valuable insights into what setting conditions tend to trigger the unwanted behaviour, and what helps it not to occur at those other times.

   e Strategic choice of the first target behaviour for recording can also re-orientate dispirited carers to see that there are still areas where the child is doing well, thus spurring them on to keep trying. The obvious behaviours to record are often those that are identified as problems. This can provide useful information, but also focuses everyone's attention on what does not appear to be going well. Consider instead the effect of focusing the child's or young person's and the carer's attention on an area where they are already enjoying success. Are they more or less likely to be motivated to tackle difficult areas later if the things they are achieving are first highlighted? And that doesn't just apply to children.

   f Although 'assessment' and 'intervention' are supposedly independent phases of the work we do with children, young people and families, judicious use of assessment tools which start to objectively reframe the situation for the family can often be an effective intervention in its own right.

3   The information presented by the client and elicited by the therapist enables a cognitive behavioural formulation to be developed, together with a working hypothesis about the presenting problem. The way in which this hypothesis is formed is described earlier in the chapter. This in turn points to the area that needs to be the focus of the CBT intervention.

4   The 'treatment' or intervention phase should start with the clinician sharing his or her working hypothesis about the nature of the problem (or diagnosis) with the client. This will generally involve a hypothesis about how and why the symptoms have arisen, together with a proposed care plan as to how they might be modified.

5   Specific cognitive behavioural techniques are then employed. The choice of this should be informed by the available evidence base, but pragmatic issues may also intervene. The range of potential interventions is broad, and the specialist CBT workforce in any single service is often very restricted.

6   Progress is usually reviewed after an agreed time or number of sessions, with the opportunity to refine or amend the working hypothesis if progress is not as anticipated.

7   Lack of a reasonable or explicable level of progress should provoke a revisiting of the formulation.

Practitioner tips for successful CBT casework

Engagement

Engage the child/young person/parents as a first priority. This does not require CBT-specific skills, and indeed it is often best to avoid narrowing down questions to 'the problem' area too soon, as you may otherwise miss out on information that could prove key to your working hypothesis. It is also important for the child/young person not to identify themselves as the problem, but rather to be able to externalize it as 'their behaviour' or 'the way they think about things'. If that is achieved, the efforts of the nurse, the client and the family can be combined against 'the problem': if not and the child feels blamed or that the difficulties are seen as inherent, it sets up an unhelpful adversarial position in which children often feel pitched against their parents, and sometimes the therapist.

Resisting pressure to put solutions before assessment

Parents and/or the young person are usually keen for an intervention to proceed as quickly as possible, as they will already have been living with the problem for some time before arriving at CAMHS. Although this is understandable, it is important for the nurse to resist the pressure to make recommendations regarding intervention before an adequate assessment has been undertaken. A useful analogy is to question how happy people would be if they took their car into a garage with a set of 'symptoms' and after five minutes of questioning the mechanic recommended that the engine be replaced, at huge cost. Would we not expect a more thorough assessment of the actual problems before we would have confidence that such expense was really necessary? Misunderstanding a young person's behavioural or emotional difficulties is also very 'expensive' for them in a number of ways. If they and their family are going to be expected to attend regular appointments, do homework tasks, complete thought records etc., it is vital that there is a clear working hypothesis and a formulation that makes a strong case for the necessity and fit of the intervention being pursued. Remember the carpenter's golden rule: *'Measure twice, cut once'!*

Focusing family resources and instilling confidence

Children and young people rarely arrive at CAMHS with a single, circumscribed difficulty. More often there will be a list of problem areas that the young person, the carers, or both want to address. It is important to resist the pressure to work on all fronts at the same time, as such efforts are likely to go the way of famous military campaigns that have committed the same error of spreading resources too thinly. Rather, it is better to agree a systematic approach in which efforts can be focused on one or perhaps two key areas initially, moving on to others once significant change has been achieved. It is also important to pick the first ones carefully. Parents may be keen to prioritize the area that is most worrying or problematic, but this may be the hardest area in which to achieve a noticeable change. In the interests of promoting morale and motivation for all involved, it is often preferable to choose an area where a 'quick win' can be expected, so that flushed with this success, it is easier to move up the hierarchy.

Predicting setbacks to lessen the impact when they arise

In most areas of health and medicine, finding that a symptom worsens after taking a supposed cure would convince you that either the diagnosis or the treatment is wrong, and that the treatment should be stopped. However, when working with behavioural problems, there is a well documented phenomenon from learning theory called the *pre-extinction burst*, in which the frequency or intensity of the behaviour targeted for change *increases* before it eventually extinguishes or significantly reduces. If parents can be forewarned of this, they can be encouraged to stay with the process through this stage, and thus reach the point where the efforts pay off. It is counter-intuitive, but by predicting the likelihood that behaviour may well worsen before it gets better, the clinician allows the carers to maintain confidence that the process is under control and going to plan, which in itself helps to contain their anxieties and maintain motivation.

It is also evident that in more cognitively-based approaches, progress rarely occurs without setbacks. Again, the therapist should anticipate this and, without being unduly negative, advise the young person that this is to be expected. Setbacks can actually be very helpful and move the therapeutic process on if clients can be assisted to *cognitively reframe* them. For example, a young person using a cognitive strategy to combat anxiety in social situations may feel initially disappointed that after 40 minutes in company, he felt it necessary to leave. This could be reframed as a very successful venture as he endured a whole 40 minutes in company (rather than taking the option of avoiding the challenge altogether). In addition, it is perhaps better to have struggled with a situation but survived it, rather than to have had a problem-free time, which might leave you waiting anxiously for 'the bubble to burst'. It is important not to dismiss the level of disappointment clients may feel regarding perceived setbacks, but also important to model for them an alternative way of evaluating their experience which does not have to reduce confidence in their capacity to change.

Summary

Cognitive-behavioural casework is rooted in sound psychological theory and now has a significant evidence base across a wide range of CAMH clinical areas. It offers a framework to inform the professional's understanding of how a child's mental health problems may have come about, what is maintaining them, and what might need to change in order for them to be successfully addressed. CBT interventions are based on individually-devised, overt and testable working hypotheses, with a focus on measurable outcomes that should indicate the success or otherwise of the intervention. A lack of success over a reasonable period triggers a re-examination of the hypothesis rather than an attribution of blame to individuals, with the potential for a new, shared understanding and intervention plan to be reached.

CBT is not a panacea for all problems, but its principles are a useful addition to the therapeutic tool-kit of the CAMH nurse.

References

Bandura, A. (1977) *Social Learning Theory*. Englewood Cliffs, NJ: Prentice-Hall.

Beck, A. (1970) Cognitive therapy: nature and relation to behaviour therapy, *Behavior Therapy*, 1(2).

Dodge, K.A. (1980) Social cognition and children's aggressive behaviour, *Child Development*, 51: 162–70.

Ellis, A. (1957) Rational psychotherapy and individual psychology, *Journal of Individual Psychology*, 13: 38–44.

Graham, P. (2005) Jack Tizard lecture: cognitive behaviour therapies for children: passing fashion or here to stay? *Child and Adolescent Mental Health*, 10(2): 57–62.

Harrington, R., Whittaker, J., Shoebridge, P. and Campbell, F. (1998) Systematic review of efficacy of cognitive behaviour therapies in child and adolescent depressive disorder, *British Medical Journal*, 316: 1559–63.

Herbert, M. (1978) *Conduct Disorders of Childhood and Adolescence: A Social Learning Perspective:* Chichester: Wiley.

Kendall, P. (1994) Treatment of anxiety disorders in children: a randomised control trial, *Journal of Consulting and Clinical Psychology*, 62: 100–10.

Kendall, P.C. and Panichelli-Mindel, S.M. (1995) Cognitive behavioural treatments, *Journal of Abnormal Child Psychology*, 23: 107–24.

King, N., Tonge, B., Heyne, D., Pritchard, M., Rollings, S., Young, D., Myerson, N. and Ollendick, T. (1998) Cognitive behavioural treatment for school-refusing children: a controlled evaluation, *Journal of the American Academy of Child and Adolescent Psychiatry*, 37: 395–403.

King, N.J., Muris, P. and Ollendick, T.H. (2005) Childhood fears and phobias: assessment and treatment, *Child and Adolescent Mental Health*, 10(2): 50–6.

March, J.S. (2005) Cognitive behavioural psychotherapy for children and adolescents with OCD: a review and recommendations for treatment, *Journal of the American Academy of Child and Adolescent Psychiatry*, 34: 7–17.

Mischel, W. (1976) *Introduction to Personality*, 2nd edn. New York: Holt, Rinehart & Winston.

Pavlov, I.P. (1927) *Conditioned Reflexes*. Oxford: Oxford University Press.

Skinner, B.F. (1938) *Science of Human Behaviour*. London: Macmillan.

Spence, S., Donovan, C. and Brechman-Toussaint, M. (2000) The treatment of childhood social phobia: the effectiveness of a social-skills training-based, cognitive behavioural intervention, with and without parental involvement, *Journal of Child Psychology and Psychiatry*, 41: 713–26.

Stallard, P. (2004) Cognitive behaviour therapy with pre-pubertal children, in P.J. Graham (ed.) *Cognitive Behaviour Therapy for Children and Families* (2nd edn). Cambridge: Cambridge University Press.

Teasdale, J.D. and Fogarty. S.J. (1979) Differential effects of induced mood on retrieval of pleasant and unpleasant events from episodic memory, *Journal of Abnormal Psychology*, 88, 248–57.

Thorndike, E.L. (1911) *Animal Intelligence: An Experimental Study of Associative Processes in Animals*, www.pstchclassics.yorku.ca.

Further reading

Graham, P. (ed.) (2005) *Cognitive Behaviour Therapy for Children and Families*, 2nd edn. Cambridge: Cambridge University Press.

Stallard, P. (2002) *Think Good, Feel Good: A Cognitive Behaviour Therapy Workbook for Children and Young People*. Chichester: Wiley.

Teasdale, J.D. and Barnard, P.J. (1993) *Affect, Cognition and Change*. Hove: Lawrence Erlbaum.

9 Nurse prescribing and medication management in CAMHS

Noreen Ryan and Teresa Norris

Key features	• The controversial use of medication within child and adolescent mental health services (CAMHS) and learning disabilities (LD).
	• Discussion of the expanding evidence base in this area and the lack of specific guidance for nurse prescribing in CAMHS.
	• The possibility of improved access to medicines for children and young people due to nurse prescribing.
	• Prescribing as one component of treatment, dependent on the undertaking of a comprehensive assessment.

Introduction

This chapter aims to provide the reader with both an understanding of the use of medication in CAMHS (including LD CAMHS), and of new ways of working for nurses in terms of independent and supplementary prescribing.

Medication management

Psycho-tropic drugs are used to treat symptoms of mental illness and are powerful agents that can change the thoughts, mood and behaviour of patients and positively impact upon their well-being and day-to-day functioning (Taylor and Thomas 2002; Callaghan and Waldcock 2006). Medicines have been used in the treatment of mental illness since the late 1940s for a range of disorders and there have been ever-advancing developments in this area (Pearson 1997). There is no doubt that the advances in therapeutic medicines have enhanced the lives of many patients. However, there are limitations to the use of medication and concerns have been expressed by patients about unwanted side-effects and an over-emphasis on medication as opposed to psycho-social interventions.

In order to safely engage in the process of nurse prescribing, a good understanding of pharmacology is required as well as clinical expertise (Cossey 2005). The use of the *British National Formulary (BNF) for Children* (BMA and Royal Pharmaceutical Society of Great Britain 2008) is an invaluable tool when considering drug interactions and reviewing recommended doses (Sutcliffe 1999; DoH 2004; BMA and Royal Pharmaceutical Society of Great Britain 2008).

The use of medicines in mental health care poses challenges to mental health nurses in terms of their role and function in the different responsibilities that they have with their patients.

There is unease about the whole issue of medication use and management by mental health nurses. However, mental health nurses have an important role to play in long-term medication management and are well placed to support patients in the use of medication.

Children and adolescents

The use of medication in the care of young people with mental health and learning disabilities is a controversial subject. Not only is the thought of using psycho-tropic medicines in this age group difficult to conceptualize, but the way these medicines work for children is not well studied, with most of the evidence for effectiveness coming from studies with adults (Fonagy et al. 2002; Smyth and Gowers 2005). It is understandable that the use of medicines with children raises issues about the long-term side-effects of medication, yet there is a lack of data and research in this area. Concerns have been raised about the impact of medication on brain development in children, therefore it is necessary to research and develop safe and effective medicines for use by children with mental health problems. It is important to ensure that children are not denied an effective intervention due to either ideological opposition or lack of knowledge about the current evidence base (Heyman and Santosh 2002).

In the UK, the use of medication in children has been more cautious than in the USA, but there has been an increase in the prescribing of medication in CAMHS over the last 30 years (Murray et al. 2004; Wong et al. 2004; Smyth and Gowers 2005). The issues of consent, capacity to make informed decisions and the legal framework surrounding the process of medication management further complicate the use of medication in children. There is a growing body of evidence that children and young people can benefit from the use of medicines in the guidance from the National Institute for Health and Clinical Excellence (NICE), in particular in relation to post-traumatic stress disorder (PTSD) (NICE 2005a); depression (NICE 2005b); obsessive-compulsive disorder (OCD) (NICE 2005c); bipolar disorder (NICE 2006a) and attention deficit hyperactivity disorder (ADHD) (NICE 2006b, 2008). This guidance offers information as to the efficacy of medication for use with children, having looked at the evidence available.

Use of medication for children with mental health problems should be just one component of a treatment package that includes psychological, social and educational interventions (Heyman and Santosh 2002; Ryan 2006; Ryan and McDougall 2009). Medications commonly used in CAMHS are listed in Table 9.1, methylphenidate hydrochloride probably being the most extensively researched drug for children (Heyman and Santosh 2002; Fonagy et al. 2002).

Table 9.1 Commonly used medications in CAMHS

Disorder	Medication
ADHD	Methylphenidate (Concerta XL; Equasym; Equasym XL; Medikinet; Ritalin)
	Atomoxetine (Straterra)
	Dexamphetamine (Dexedrine)
Depression	Fluoxetine (Prozac)
OCD	Sertraline
Tourette syndrome	Clonidine
	Sulpiride
	Risperidone
Psychosis	Atypical antipsychotics
	• Risperidone
	• Olanzapine
Sleep	Melatonin

The use of medication in CAMHS and LD is well established and it is acknowledged that psycho-social and psycho-pharmacological interventions are used to improve day-to-day functioning for children. Prescribing medication has previously been the domain of medical colleagues with mental health and LD nurses playing a supportive role in medication management. However, the modernization of the National Health Service (NHS) and the introduction of non-medical prescribing (referred to as 'nurse prescribing') has had a profound impact on the roles and responsibilities of mental health and LD nurses, and nurse prescribing will no doubt continue to evolve (Dimond 2003; Bradley and Nolan 2005; O'Dowd 2007; Snowden 2007; McDougall and Ryan 2008; Ryan and McDougall 2009).

Nurse prescribing

History

Nurse prescribing began by giving nurses the right to prescribe a limited range of products to patients in order to speed up access to medicines (DoH 1986). Since then, the scope, practice and competence of nurse prescribing has continued to develop with the publication of the Crown Reports (DoH 1989, 1999). In May 2006 the nurses' extended formulary for independent prescribing was changed to include most licensed medications within the BNF for conditions within their clinical competency (DoH 2006). The legal framework around nurse prescribing continues to evolve and be updated.

Education and competencies required

In order to have the competence, skills and knowledge to be an independent and/or supplementary nurse prescriber, nurses are required to undertake independent, extended and supplementary prescribing training. Requirements for nurse prescribing training and education include the ability to study at degree level, and at least three years of post-registration clinical nursing experience. At least one year's clinical experience immediately preceding the training should be in the clinical area in which they intend to prescribe.

It is necessary for nurses to be able to assimilate all aspects of their training in order to assess the presenting condition, understand the patient's individual circumstances and have sufficient knowledge about the medicines to become a proficient and competent prescriber (DoH 2006). It is important to acknowledge that not all nurses will be required to become prescibers as roles vary between NHS organizations. In order for mental health and LD nurses to take up the responsibilities of nurse prescribing it is necessary for them to have a good understanding of psycho-pharmacology that will assist them in their prescribing decisions (Robson and Gray 2007).

Nurse prescribing in mental health

The UK government has introduced new ways of working for mental health nurses and psychiatrists that aim to expand patient access to health care and to improve outcomes for patients (DoH 2007). Much nurse prescribing experience in mental health comes from the USA (Nolan *et al.* 2001) and prior to its introduction in the UK the prescribing of medicines followed a well-established and familiar pattern: the doctor assesses the patient, makes a diagnosis and recommends treatment which, if a medicine, the pharmacist dispenses for administration by either the patient or the nurse. With the introduction of new ways of working this process has been dramatically changed (Bailey and Hemingway 2006).

There are mental health nurses who see nurse prescribing as a clear improvement in patient care due to their having closer working relationships with their patients and therefore being in a better position to recognize side-effects and act quickly to moderate these, thus avoiding poor health outcomes. Conversely, mental health nurses who oppose the introduction of nurse prescribing are concerned that this task moves the focus of intervention away from the core nursing roles (e.g. psycho-social care and psycho-therapeutic conversations). Some nurses fear that the process of prescribing will alter their therapeutic relationship with their patients (Nolan and Badger 2000). There is concern that nurses do not in any case pay enough attention to the basics of mental health nursing care without the introduction of other tasks and responsibilities (Castledine 2004; Keen 2006).

The scope of nurse prescribing in CAMHS

Approximately a quarter of the CAMHS workforce consists of nursing personnel (Audit Commission 1999). Nurse prescribing has been a developing concept in the NHS for over 20 years (DoH 1986, 1989, 1999; Jones *et al.* 2005; Skingsley *et al.* 2006) and it is anticipated that the formal introduction of nurse prescribing will have a dramatic effect on the role of CAMH and LD nurses. Currently, the implementation of nurse prescribing in CAMHS has been in relation to the treatment and management of children with LD, where often psycho-social interventions are difficult to deliver, and ADHD, particularly where medicines are considered to be first-line interventions (NICE 2006b, 2008). However, independent and supplementary nurse prescribing can be developed and implemented more widely within CAMHS for the care and treatment of children with a range of mental disorders including depression and anxiety-based disorders such as OCD (Ryan 2007a).

As previously stated, good practice recommends the use of psycho-pharmacological interventions as part of a wider treatment package. However, there are general concerns about the use of medicines by children that go beyond nurse prescribing (Heyman and Santosh 2002; Smyth and Gowers 2005; Ryan 2007a). It is a general principle of good practice that children, adolescents and their families should be supported to make decisions about medicines based on sound information regarding the relative risks and benefits. However, in the UK there is a lack of good evidence of effectiveness from randomized controlled trials. Much of the evidence for the use of medicines with children comes from the USA where diagnostic and research criteria are different. Despite the lack of evidence on the short- and long-term outcomes, there has been a dramatic increase in the use of medicines by children in recent years. A UK study has shown that of nine countries, including the USA, Canada and other European states, the UK is responsible for the highest increase of prescribing for children (Wong *et al.* 2004).

Efficacy and safety

The efficacy and safety of medicines in adult populations cannot automatically be assumed to apply to children. Indeed, the majority of medicines used with children in the UK are only licensed for use with people over 18 years of age. They are tested for efficacy and safety with adult populations and children are excluded from the trials. An independent nurse prescriber can prescribe medications for uses that are outside of the product licence of those drugs, within their range of knowledge and expertise. The Nursing and Midwifery Council (NMC) issued standards regarding this in 2006, in line with those of the General Medical Council (GMC), and had previously stated that 'this use of medication is most likely to be the case when prescribing medication for children' (NMC 2006: 29). According to the World Health Organization (WHO) (2004: 21) 'Informed use of unlicensed and off licensed use of medication is deemed to be necessary in paediatric practice' and this is supported by the National Service Framework (NSF) for children in relation to medication management (DoH 2004).

Special considerations for nurse prescribing in LD and CAMHS

Specific guidance regarding medication management for children with LD is limited and a high proportion of studies are carried out within the adult population. The incidence of children with LD developing mental illness or problem behaviour is significantly higher than in the general population. Figures show that between 40 and 50 per cent of such children are likely to develop significant psychiatric illness (Lask *et al.* 2003; Bhaumik and Brandford 2005). Overall it is estimated that 30–70 per cent of children with LD (depending upon the level of LD) present with mental illnesses that are representative of a broad range of disorders, but unfortunately a great many go undiagnosed due to a lack of recognition by professionals. Reasons for non-identification of mental health problems in children with LD include misconceptions that symptoms exhibited are related to the LD or the symptoms present non-specifically or atypically and are not considered significant. This picture is further complicated by the presence comorbid difficulties (Lask *et al.* 2003).

In view of these difficulties in diagnosing complex issues, an assessment is best carried out by professionals who are experienced in the field of LD, behavioural difficulties and mental disorders. Due to the complexity of determining the aetiology of many symptoms presented by children with LD, historically there has been, and still is, concern regarding the excessive and inappropriate use of psycho-tropic medications (Taylor *et al.* 2005).

When considering the use of medication within LD, clarification of the rationale for treatment, the impact of medication, possible adverse effects and interactions with other medications (especially anti-convulsants) should be sought (Taylor *et al.* 2005). Due to developmental problems it is difficult to gain feedback directly from children and it is necessary to communicate with parents, carers and teachers to obtain relevant information about changes in behaviours that have been targeted by medication. Often patients will not comply with the monitoring regime and so the ability to identify adverse effects is imperative. Due to the input already provided by the nurse prescriber, and the relationship built up with the child and their family/carers in the assessment process, it is more likely that this can be achieved.

Nurse prescribing in LD is more complex than in CAMHS, although it follows the same principles. Most children with LD will use behaviours as a form of communication. Therefore, when prescribing for these children it is important to remember that many will not respond in a predictable way. Idiosyncratic reaction and extreme adverse effects are commonplace and it is safer to commence medication at a much lower dose than recommended and to proceed slowly and cautiously (WHO 2004). Often in the presence of comorbidity it is necessary to target symptoms rather than diagnosis. Longer trial times may be necessary before improvements are noted. It is advisable to make only one change at a time, whether this be medication or other treatments, so as to avoid confusion as to which has brought about improvements or deterioration (Taylor *et al.* 2005). It is likely that a higher percentage of medication used within LD is prescribed off-licence. For ethical reasons there is a significant lack of clinical trials involving patients with LD and so use in LD cannot be included in the licence. Much information comes from studies and reports regarding the use of medications' off-licence use by doctors nationally and internationally (Riddle *et al.* 1999).

The prescribing processes

The assessment process is pivotal to the consideration of prescribing, with prescribing being only part of a package of assessment and intervention (Eminson 2005). Nursing assessment is the cornerstone of influencing prescribing decisions. Without a comprehensive assessment it is unsafe to consider prescribing in any circumstances, as a diagnosis and formulation of the difficulties has not been made and therefore interventions cannot begin to be considered.

Reaching a formulation and diagnosis

Having considered all the information gained through the assessment process and in discussion with the parents/carers and, where appropriate, the child or adolescent, formulation, diagnosis and intervention can begin to be negotiated. Interventions for the treatment of disorders in CAMHS and LD are varied and a multi-modal approach is often required. Nurses should consider the following as part of the treatment package:

- psycho-educational measures;
- psycho-social interventions (e.g. cognitive behavioural therapy – CBT), family therapy, parent training and behavioural interventions, school-based behavioural interventions and psycho-educational interventions);
- psycho-pharmacological interventions.

Nurse prescribing

If the use of medication is thought to be an appropriate intervention the principles of prescribing in CAMHS are the same as those to be considered by any prescribing nurse. Prescribing should be applied in the context of a comprehensive assessment and care plan and in collaboration with medical colleagues (McDougall and Ryan 2008). Nurses can use tools such as the 'prescribing pyramid' to inform prescribing decisions. The pyramid provides seven principles of safe prescribing (NPC 1999). Ryan (2007b) and Ryan and McDougall (2009) have illustrated the use of the prescribing pyramid for prescribing in one aspect of CAMHS – ADHD. The steps on the pyramid are as follows:

1 *The patient* – consider the specific needs of the child or young person, taking into account any medicines already prescribed, including over-the-counter and herbal preparations.
2 *Which strategy* – other treatment options should be considered as prescribing a medicine may not be the most appropriate action.
3 *Choice of product* – what is the evidence base for the product to be used (e.g. NICE guidance, consideration of drug interactions, comorbid difficulties, child and family choice, concerns regarding concordance and safety of medicines)?
4 *Negotiate a contract* – use of independent or supplementary prescribing and agreement with the child, parents or carers.
5 *Review the patient* – review is important to assess the usefulness of treatment and also to manage unwanted effects.
6 *Keeping records* – all nurses are required to keep detailed records and in terms of prescribing, consent and efficacy issues.
7 *Reflection* – continued development, clinical supervision and reflection on practice is essential to competent nurse prescribing.

Heyman and Santosh (2002) and Fonagy *et al.* (2002) provide reflective questions for nurses to ask when considering prescribing (see Box 9.1).

> **Box 9.1 Reflective questions when considering prescribing**
>   • Does this condition have an evidence base for medication use?
>   • Are the symptoms of the disorder severe and causing impairment sufficient to consider medication management?
>   • What behaviours are to be targeted and improved by the medication?
>   • What are the risks versus the benefits of treatment in the short and long term?
>   • How will progress and outcomes be monitored and reviewed in collaboration between the prescriber, child or young person and their family?

Nurse prescribing in practice

Nurse prescribers can engage in two types of prescribing:

1 independent;
2 supplementary.

Independent prescribing is described as follows:

> that the prescriber takes responsibility for the clinical assessment of the patient, establishing a diagnosis and the clinical management required, as well as for the prescribing where necessary and the appropriateness of any prescriptions.
>
> (DoH 2003: 12)

While it is not a requirement to have a clinical management plan (CMP) for independent prescribing, it is felt to be good practice to have a plan in place, drawn up with patient or carers, and independent prescibers are using an adaptation of the CMP format for this.

Supplementary prescribing is designed to maximize the benefits for the patient. It allows the patient to be involved in the decision-making process about who prescribes and manages the medication, is helpful for management of chronic conditions and permits flexible use of the workforce (Shuttle 2004; Beckwith and Franklin 2007). Therefore, supplementary prescribing is defined as:

> a voluntary prescribing partnership between an independent prescriber (IP) (doctor) and a supplementary prescriber (SP) (nurse or pharmacist), to implement an agreed patient specific CMP with the patient's agreement.
>
> (DoH 2003: 8)

The CMP is drawn up jointly between the independent and supplementary prescibers, clearly stating the indications for treatment, aims and medications to be prescribed by the supplementary prescriber on a named patient basis. There are regular reviews between the independent and supplementary prescribers regarding the progress of the treatment and the CMP is reviewed at least annually and altered/ended as necessary. There are no restrictions to the clinical conditions that a supplementary nurse prescriber can treat, but a CMP needs to be negotiated between the patient, and the independent and supplementary prescribers (Jones 2006; Barlow *et al.* 2008). Supplementary prescribing is beneficial to prescribing unlicensed medicines, and for controlled drugs that cannot be prescribed by independent prescribers (Beckwith and Franklin 2007).

It has been suggested that for children with mental health problems and LD the implementation of supplementary and independent nurse prescribing will provide care that is timelier, will reduce delays in initiating treatment and allow nurses to titrate doses and stop one medication and commence another (DoH 2005).

Box 9.2 Case scenario: Paul

Paul, aged 7, is referred to CAMHS following concerns expressed by his parents and teachers about his social and academic progress in school. Paul was finding it hard to sustain friendships and appeared to be an unpopular child. He was falling behind his peers with his school work.

Comprehensive CAMHS assessment formulated that Paul had significant impairing symptoms of hyperactivity, inattention and impulsivity, reaching criteria for ADHD. There were no other family or developmental issues that could account for the pre-senting symptoms. He did not have learning needs and was well supported by his parents and extended family.

The evidence-based interventions offered were:

1 psycho-education;
2 psycho-social intervention (parenting and behavioural management);
3 pharmacology.

Paul, his parents and his school were given information about ADHD so that they were able to understand his difficulties. Paul's parents engaged in sessions to look at man-aging aspects of his behaviour. However, they continued to feel that Paul was not making progress in terms of friends or school work and he remained very hyperactive. They therefore opted for a trial of medication.

Pharmacology

1 Is there an evidence-based medication?
   • Yes: methylphenidate and atomoxetine.
2 Are the symptoms of the disorder causing impairment?
   • Yes, in terms of Paul's family relationships, behaviour, peer relationships and academic progress.
3 What behaviours are to be targeted?
   • Hyperactivity.
   • Inattention.
   • Impulsivity.
4 What are the risks versus the benefits of treatment?
   • Unwanted effects of treatment are concerns about appetite, sleep, feeling sad and tearful, headaches and stomach aches. Potential longer-term difficulties with increased blood pressure and pulse, and slowed growth have been identified.
   • The known risks of methylphenidate and atomoxetine have been studied. Some young people are unable to tolerate unwanted effects and do not continue. There is little data detailing the long-term effects of treatment.
   • What is known is that if the impairment in social and academic functioning caused by ADHD is not treated then young people will have poor outcomes in terms of academic achievement, will be more likely to be involved in crime, will have poor work histories and relationship failure, and more mental health prob-lems in adult life.
   • NICE have made the following recommendations about medications for ADHD:

     i. the presence of comorbid conditions (e.g. tic disorders, Tourette's syndrome, epilepsy);

    ii the different adverse effects of the drugs;

    iii specific issues regarding compliance identified for the individual child or adolescent, for example, problems created by the need to administer a midday treatment dose at school;

    iv the potential for drug diversion (where the medication is forwarded on to others for non-prescription uses) and/or misuse;

    v the preferences of the child/adolescent and/or his or her parent or guardian.

5 What monitoring will be undertaken?

- Health screening including cardiovascular review.
- Height, weight, blood pressure and pulse.
- Symptom checklist.
- Side-effects questionnaires.
- The trial of medication will be reviewed with Paul, his parents and his teachers to establish its effectiveness.

6 What type of nurse prescribing (independent or supplementary)?

- Methylphenidate supplementary prescribing.
- Atomoxetine independent prescribing.

Pharmacology

Is a medicine evidence-based	• Methylphenidate (supplementary prescribing) • Atomoxetine (independent prescribing)
What behaviours are to be targeted	• Hyperactivity • Inattention • Impulsivity
What monitoring will take place	• Physical health and cardiovascular review: height, weight, blood pressure and pulse • Effectiveness of symptom reduction without unwanted effects of medication

Decisions

Paul's parents opted for a trial of atomoxetine rather than methylphenidate as they were concerned about giving Paul an amphetamine-based medicine. Atomoxetine can be prescribed independently by appropriately qualified nurses and a dose calculation is required, determined by body weight. This trial of non-stimulant treatment was unsuccessful in terms of reducing hyperactivity, impulsivity and inattention and Paul's parents agreed to a trial of methylphenidate. Currently, methylphenidate can only be prescribed on a supplementary basis by suitably qualified nurses and is commenced at a low dose three times a day and increased in line with the doses in the children's BNF as long as unwanted effects are not experienced. The trial of methylphenidate helped to reduce hyperactivity, impulsivity and improve concentration at home and school, where Paul was reported to remain in his seat, follow the lesson, work independently, produce more and better quality work. He also appeared to be more sociable with and accepted by his peer group.

Routine review

Paul had a positive response to medication without side-effects but requires routine review of the treatment effects and his physical health (height, weight, blood pressure and pulse). Paul is growing and gaining weight appropriately. His parents are pleased with his progress and have made changes to their parenting approaches to Paul. As a result family relationships have improved.

What safeguards need to be in place?

With the extension of nurses' roles in supplementary prescribing and a movement away from traditional nursing practice, clear frameworks to review the process of nurse prescribing need to be introduced within NHS Trust clinical governance structures (Jones and Harbone 2005). The recent publication of the *BNF for Children* in 2008 provides invaluable support and information about prescribing for children (BMA and Royal Pharmaceutical Society of Great Britain 2008). There are a number of important general considerations when prescribing for children. These include:

- Children metabolize medicines at different rates to adults, therefore special precautions should be taken when prescribing, taking into account age, weight, dose calculations and the developmental status of the child (Sutcliffe 1999; Beckwith and Franklin 2007; BMA and Royal Pharmaceutical Society of Great Britain 2008).
- Concordance with treatment by the child, adolescent and their family or carer is vital and needs to be established by the nurse.
- The nurse must assess the ability of the child or adolescent to take care of their own medication, and address issues related to supervision and safety of medicines in the home.
- Depending on the age and wishes of the child or adolescent, they, as well as their family or carers, should be involved in the decision-making process. This may cause some difficulties when prescribing for children with LD who, after the age of 16, will need to be assessed regarding their competency under the Mental Capacity Act (DoH 2005).

Continued professional development (CPD)

Nurses are required to maintain their own competence and declare that they have met standards of practice and study in order to retain their nursing registration with the NMC (NMC 2004; Hobden 2007). Nurse prescribers are not expected to undertake extra CPD, but highlight prescribing practice as part of their CPD needs. They are required to demonstrate competency with assessments and carry out prescribing decisions regularly, and reflection should be occur within the context of the multi-disciplinary team (NMC 2008). Clinical supervision is an integral part of CPD and nurses can use this to maintain competence (Armstrong 2006; Ryan 2007b).

Challenges associated with nurse prescribing

The challenges and opportunities of nurse prescribing in CAMHS and LD are evident in that it changes the therapeutic relationship between the nurse, doctor and their patient. Not all nurses will want, or be required to, become nurse prescribers, and not all CAMHS services will want to develop non-medical prescribing. It is important to ensure that nurses continue to be bound by their professional code of conduct when implementing nurse prescribing, the core values being that we 'do good and do not harm', we involve children and young people in the process of obtaining consent to treatment and we provide information accurately, truthfully and understandably (NMC 2004). The pace of change in mental health nurse prescribing has been slow. However, the Department of Health is considering extending the boundaries of nurse prescribing in mental health, CAMHS and LD and there will almost certainly be further developments in the future.

Service users accept the change in practice of mental health and LD nurses prescribing rather than doctors, and the benefits reported by service users in relation to non-medical prescribing are many (Harrison 2003; Wix 2007). These include improved access to medicines, reduced waiting times for prescriptions, more freedom of choice, and greater flexibility and responsiveness. Further research into the risks, benefits and outcomes of medication use in CAMHS and LD and the implementation of non-medical prescribing is nevertheless required.

Summary

The introduction of nurse prescribing offers the promise of improved access to medicines for children and young people in CAMHS and LD. Independent and supplementary prescribing are 'new ways of working' for nurses, however, processes need to be in place to ensure competent practice and safety for patients. Nurse prescribing needs to take into account individual nurses' training, expertise and competence to ensure patient safety and choice at all times. CPD and clinical supervision will allow nurses to keep their knowledge up to date, be aware of changes to legislation and maintain their level of competency.

Finally, you may wish to attempt the reflective questions given in Box 9.3.

Box 9.3 Reflective questions

- When would you consider use of a psycho-tropic medicine appropriate?
- Put yourself in the position of a parent making a decision about the use of medication for their child. What information would you need in order to make an informed decision? What information would you provide?
- When discussing medication management with children and adolescents, do you listen to the views of the young person as well as the parents/carers?
- Do nurses have a role in the prescribing of medication in CAMHS and LD?
- Does nurse prescribing in CAMHS improve quality of care?
- Is there an expectation that all nurses in CAMHS and LD train to be nurse prescribers and what competencies, training and support would you require to take up this role?

References

Armstrong, M. (2006) Self-harm, young people and nursing, in T. McDougall (ed.) *Child and Adolescent Mental Health Nursing*. London: Blackwell.

Audit Commission (1999) *Children in Mind: Child and Adolescent Mental Health Services*. London: Audit Commission.

Bailey, K.P. and Hemingway, S. (2006) Psychiatric/mental health nurses as non-medical prescribers: validating their role in the prescribing process, in J.R. Cutliffe and M.F. Ward (eds) *Key Debates in Psychiatric and Mental Health Nursing*. Edinburgh: Churchill Livingstone, Elsevier.

Barlow, M., Magorrain, K., Jones, M. and Edwards, K. (2008) Nurse prescribing in an Alzheimer's disease service: a reflective account, *Mental Health Practice*, 11(7): 32–5.

Beckwith, S. and Franklin, P. (2007) *Oxford Handbook of Nurse Prescribing*. Oxford: Oxford University Press.

Bhaumik, S. and Branford, D. (2005) *The Frith Prescribing Guidelines for Adults with Learning Disability*. Abingdon: Taylor & Francis.

BMA (British Medical Association) and Royal Pharmaceutical Society of Great Britain (2008) *BNF for Children*. London: BMJ Publications.

Bradley, E. and Nolan, P. (2005) Non-medical prescribing and mental health nursing: prominent issues, *Mental Health Practice*, 8(5): 16–19.

Callaghan, P. and Waldcock, H. (2006) *Oxford Handbook of Mental Health Nursing*. Oxford: Oxford University Press.

Castledine, G. (2004) Basic nursing principles need to be remembered, *British Journal of Nursing*, 13(6): 343.

Cossey, M. (2005). Applied pharmacology, in M. Courtenay and M. Griffiths (eds) *Independent and Supplementary Prescribing: An Essential Guide*. Cambridge: Cambridge University Press.

Dimond, B. (2003) The introduction of nurse prescribing 2: final Crown Report, *British Journal of Nursing*, 12(16): 980–3.

DoH (Department of Health) (1986) *Nursing: A Focus for Care. Report of the Community Nursing Review. The Cumberledge Report*. London: DHSS.

DoH (Department of Health) (1989) *Report for the Advisory Group on Nurse Prescribing (Crown Report)*. London. HMSO.

DoH (Department of Health) (1999) *Review of Prescribing, Supply and Administration of Medicines: Final Report (Crown Review)*. London. HMSO.

DoH (Department of Health) (2003) *Supplementary Prescribing by Nurses and Pharmacists within the NHS in England: A Guide for Implementation*. London: HMSO.

DoH (Department of Health) (2004) *National Service Framework for Children, Young People and Maternity Services: Standard 10, Medicines for Children and Young People*. London: HMSO.

DoH (Department of Health) (2005) *Mental Capacity Act*. London: HMSO.

DoH (Department of Health) (2006) *Improving Patients' Access to Medicines: A Guide to Implementing Nurse and Pharmacist Independent Prescribing in the NHS in England*. London: HMSO.

DoH (Department of Health) (2007) *New Ways of Working for Everyone: Developing and Sustaining a Capable and Flexible Workforce*. London: HMSO.

Eminson, M. (2005) Assessment in child and adolescent psychiatry, in S. Gowers (ed.) *Seminars in Child and Adolescent Psychiatry*, 2nd edn. Royal College of Psychiatrists. London: Gaskell.

Fonagy, P., Target, M., Cottrell, D., Phillips, J. and Kurtz, Z. (2002) *What Works for Whom? A Critical Review of Treatments for Children and Adolescents*. London: Guilford Press.

Harrison, A. (2003) Mental health service users' views of nurse prescribing, *Nurse Prescribing*, 1(2): 78–85.

Heyman, I. and Santosh, P. (2002) Pharmacological and other physical treatments, in M. Rutter and E. Taylor (eds) *Child and Adolescent Psychiatry*, 4th edn. Oxford: Blackwell.

Hobden, A. (2007) Continuing professional development for nurse prescribers, *Nurse Prescribing*, 5(4): 153–5.

Jones, A. (2006) Supplementary prescribing: relationships between nurses and psychiatrists on hospital psychiatric wards, *Journal of Psychiatric and Mental Health Nursing*, 13: 3–11.

Jones, A. and Harbone, G. (2005) Supplementary prescribing in hospital settings. *Mental Health Practice*, 9(1): 38–40.

Jones, A., Doyle, V., Pyke, S. and Harborne, G. (2005) New roles for nurses and psychiatrists in the management of long-term conditions, *Mental Health Practice*, 9(3): 16–20.

Keen, T. (2006) Gently applying the brakes to the beguiling allure of P/MH nurse prescribing, in S.P. Thomas and A. Sheehan (eds) *Key Debates in Psychiatric and Mental Health Nursing*. London: Churchill Livingstone, Elsevier.

Lask, B., Taylor, S. and Nunn, K. (2003) *Practical Child Psychiatry: The Clinicians Guide*. London: BMJ Publishing.

McDougall, T. and Ryan, N. (2008). Nurse prescribing in the UK: invited commentary, *Journal of Child and Adolescent Psychiatric Nursing* (accepted for publication).

Murray, M.L., de Vries, C.S. and Wong, I.C.K. (2004) A drug utilisation study of antidepressants in children and adolescents using the General Practice Research Database, *Archives of Disease in Childhood*, 89: 1098–102.

NICE (National Institute for Health and Clinical Excellence) (2005a) *Post-traumatic Stress Disorder (PTSD): The Management of PTSD in Adults and Children in Primary and Secondary Care*. London: NCCMH.

NICE (National Institute for Health and Clinical Excellence) (2005b) *Depression in Children and Young People: Identification and Management in Primary, Community and Secondary Care*, Clinical Guideline 28. London: NICE.

NICE (National Institute for Health and Clinical Excellence) (2005c) *Obsessive Compulsive Disorder: Core Interventions in the Treatment of Obsessive Compulsive Disorder and Body Dysmorphic Disorder*, Clinical Guideline 31. London: NICE.

NICE (National Institute for Health and Clinical Excellence) (2006a) *Bipolar Disorder: The Management of Bipolar Disorder in Adults and Adolescents in Primary and Secondary Care*. London: NICE.

NICE (National Institute for Health and Clinical Excellence) (2006b). *Methylphenidate, Atomoxetine and Dexamfetamine for Attention Deficit Hyperactivity Disorder (ADHD) in Children and Adolescents*, Review of Technology Appraisal 13. London: NICE.

NICE (National Institute for Health and Clinical Excellence) (2008) *Attention Deficit Hyperactivity Disorder: Diagnosis and Management of ADHD in Children, Young People and Adults*, Clinical Guideline 72. London: NCCMH.

NMC (Nursing and Midwifery Council) (2004) *The NMC Code of Professional Conduct, Performance and Ethics*. London: NMC.

NMC (Nursing and Midwifery Council) (2006) *Standards of Proficiency for Nurse and Midwife Prescribers – Protecting the Public through Professional Standards*. London: NMC.

NMC (Nursing and Midwifery Council) (2008) *Guidance for Continuing Professional Development for Nurse and Midwife Prescribers*, Circular 10/2008. London: NMC.

Nolan, P. and Badger, F. (2000) Mental health nurse prescribing: added chore or golden opportunity? *Mental Health Practice*, 4(1): 12–15.

Nolan, P., Can, N. and Harold, L. (2001) Mental health nurse prescribing: the US experience, *Mental Health Practice*, 4(8): 4–7.

NPC (National Prescribing Centre) (1999) Signposts for prescribing nurses – general principles of good prescribing, *Nurse Prescribing Bulletin*, 1(1): 1–4.

O'Dowd, A. (2007) The power to prescribe, *Nursing Times*, 103(3): 16–18.

Pearson, G.S. (1997) Psychopharmacology, in B. Schoen Johnson (ed.) *Adaptation and Growth: Psychiatric-Mental Health Nursing*, 4th edn. Philadelphia, PA: Lippincott.

Riddle, M.A, Kastelic, E.A. and Frosch, E. (1999) Pediatric psychopharmacology, *Journal of Child Psychology and Psychiatry*, 41(1): 73–90.

Robson, D. and Gray, R. (2007) Prescribing psychotropic medication: what nurses need to know, *Nurse Prescribing*, 5(4): 148–52.

Ryan, N. (2006) Nursing children and young people with attention deficit hyperactivity disorder (ADHD), in T. McDougall (ed.) *Child and Adolescent Mental Health Nursing*. London: Blackwell.

Ryan, N. (2007a) Non medical prescribing in a child and adolescent mental health service, *Mental Health Practice*, 11(1): 40–4.

Ryan, N. (2007b) Nurse prescribing in child and adolescent mental health services, *Mental Health Practice*, 10(10): 35–7.

Ryan, N. and McDougall, T. (2009) *Nursing Children and Young People with ADHD*. London: Routledge.

Shuttle, B. (2004) Non-medical prescribing in a multidisciplinary team context, in M. Courtenay and

M. Griffiths (eds) *Independent and Supplementary Prescribing: An Essential Guide*. Cambridge: Greenwich Medical Media.

Skingsley, D., Bradley, E.J. and Nolan, P. (2006) Neuropharmacology and mental health nurse prescribers, *Journal of Clinical Nursing*, 15: 989–97.

Smyth, B. and Gowers, S.G. (2005) Principles of treatment, service delivery and psychopharmacology, in S. Gowers (ed.) *Seminars in Child and Adolescent Psychiatry*, 2nd edn. London Royal College of Psychiatrists.

Snowden, A. (2007) Why mental health nurses should prescribe, *Nurse Prescribing*, 5(6): 193–8.

Sutcliffe, A. (1999) Prescribing medicines for children, *British Medical Journal*, 319: 70–1.

Taylor, D. and Thomas, B. (2002) in B. Thomas, S. Hardy and P. Cutting (eds) *Stuart and Sundeen's Mental Health Nursing Principles and Practice*. London: Mosby.

Taylor, D., Paton, C. and Kerwin, R. (2005) *2005–2006 Prescribing Guidelines*, 8th edn. Abingdon: Taylor & Francis.

WHO (World Health Organization) (2004) *Guide to Mental and Neurological Health in Primary Care. A Guide to Mental and Neurological Ill Health in Adults, Adolescents and Children*, 2nd edn. London: Royal Society of Medicine Press.

Wix, S. (2007) Independent nurse prescribing in the mental health setting, *Nursing Times*, 103(44): 30–1.

Wong, I.C.K., Murray, M.L., Camilleri-Novak, D. and Stephens, P. (2004) Increased prescribing trends of paediatric psychotropic medications, *Archives of Disease of Childhood*, 89: 1131–2.

Inpatient **CAMH** nursing: two different models of care

Sarah Hogan, Ged Rogers and Neil Hemstock

> **Key features**
> - Outline of a therapeutic community.
> - Outline of an acute inpatient unit.
> - Outline of the differences and similarities between the two models.

Introduction

The purpose of this chapter is to capture some of the elements of how nurses can make a valuable contribution to young people's care when they are admitted to an inpatient unit. The chapter begins with the nursing role in a therapeutic community model of inpatient care. There is then a description of an acute unit. The range of tasks undertaken by staff in any inpatient unit is discussed. The key issue of staff dynamics is also explored. At the end of the chapter we invite you to reflect on the similarities and differences between the two models.

Inpatient provision: therapeutic community model

Child and adolescent mental health (CAMH) nurses have a major role to play in treatment programmes where they use specialist skills in establishing therapeutic relationships conducive to intensive assessment and intervention (Killeen 1990). The development and management of the therapeutic milieu is seen as a role unique to nurses (Butterworth 1991). Yet, the literature on the importance of their role in the care of mentally distressed adolescents and its place within the continuum of child and adolescent mental health services (CAMHS) provision is sparse. In this section we explore elements of this specialist intervention through an examination of the nurse/client relationship within inpatient settings. We suggest that therapeutic relationships can best be established through a collaborative process that occurs within an environmentally managed therapeutic milieu.

Developing a therapeutic milieu in inpatient settings

The purpose of providing a therapeutic milieu is to structure the adolescent's daily life experience in such a way that everything that they experience has therapeutic potential. In other words, milieu treatment uses the environment and relationships developed within that environment to improve the young person's mental health (Rowe 1988). Milieu treatment/therapy is a form of systematic environmental support, a powerful treatment used since the early 1950s. Gunderson (1978) describes a conceptual framework for milieu management that includes five therapeutic variables that are essential for the establishment and maintenance of the milieu:

- containment;
- structure;
- support;
- involvement;
- validation.

These variables are discussed briefly.

Containment

The function of containment is to maintain the safety of individuals, promoting physical well-being when the adolescent struggles to regain and maintain self-control. The containment does not need to be rigid and regimented but can have a degree of flexibility to meet the needs of individuals within the community. However, it is important that the adolescents are aware of the rules of the milieu environment and the consequences of not adhering to these. At times all adolescents will test rules and it is equally important that nurses respond in a firm but fair, calm and sensitive manner, demonstrating an acceptance and understanding towards the individuals while being competent in their duty to gain control and offer the adolescents the security that they require. Adolescents need to continue to develop a sense of their own autonomy, and to learn that when they test limits or demonstrate lack of self-control, others will need to intervene for the safety of the individual and others. Adolescents in inpatient settings need to feel reassured that the nurses will provide safety and containment and accept the adolescent's dependency without investing in control for the sake of it.

Structure

Structure is the process by which activities and time schedules are organized within the unit. The structure allows for the organization of time, place and person within the milieu. Behaviours that are predictable and repetitive carry psychological benefits for adolescents who may be in mental health crisis or traumatized as a result of early life experiences. Such young people may have difficulties managing their arousal patterns and emotional regulation. Thus, when there is a structure to daily life the young person is able to focus on modifying and building more appropriate psychological responses. In the same way that adolescents are familiar with the rules of the environment it is equally important for them to be familiar with the daily structure of the unit and nurses should ensure that the daily routines are adhered to and that young people are aware of what is expected of them.

Support

The aim of providing support is to attempt to build the adolescents' self-esteem by offering them an environment that reduces anxiety and enables them to feel secure. In such an environment the adolescents have an opportunity to move beyond a trusting relationship, and to gain mastery over more mature developmental tasks. Adolescents with mental health difficulties and traumatic histories may have been brought up in chaotic environments where the accomplishment of psychological tasks has not been validated and therefore they learn to adapt using maladaptive strategies such as dissociation and identification with aggressors. Such strategies may have served them well within a chaotic environment, but they are not useful in a nurturing environment such as milieu therapy. Thus, the adolescents become 'stuck' in a particular developmental stage, unable to mobilize personal resources for moving forward (Berliner and Lipovsky 1992). To ensure that the inpatient setting remains therapeutic the nurse needs to reflect appropriate behaviour and mastery over developmental tasks in a genuine and respectful style. Acceptance of the adolescents, validation of their feelings and attending to what they are communicating conveys such a supportive approach.

It is important for nurses working within the therapeutic milieu to be aware of how individual adolescents relate to individual members of the multi-disciplinary team. Understanding of concepts such as transference and projection is essential. Most adolescents will make some effort to engage in normal developmental activities in a nurturing environment, and support can be offered through discussion about social issues, feedback on accomplishment of physical or psychological tasks or success in social or peer relationships. Such accomplishments demonstrate both an improvement in self-esteem and collaboration within the milieu therapy.

Involvement

Gunderson (1978: 330) describes involvement as 'the process which causes patients to attend actively to their social environment and interact with it'. Within the inpatient setting young people have to relate both to their peers and to the professionals working within the environment. When the therapeutic milieu offers time to reflect on behaviours and situations, young people are able to use the group as a reference point for their own behaviours and interactions. While fostering an approach that is focused on helping oneself and others through the community processes, it also provides an opportunity for safely testing responses to new interactions and behaviours. Nurses can act as positive role models to intervene to buffer tensions, help navigate rules and resolve conflicts within the peer group situation. They can support adolescents through this process by involving them in discussions and reflections on the maladaptive behaviours and suggesting interpretations about their need to act in this manner based on their symptoms or their earlier history. This can be done within the community group or within individual sessions, to provide the adolescent with an opportunity to explore their maladaptive behaviour from a number of perspectives to be able to address issues more appropriately in the future.

Validation

Validation enables adolescents to understand the connections between their thoughts, emotions and behaviour, and to learn to reflect in order to develop self-enhancing, rather than self-destructive, behaviours. Creating opportunities for adolescents to relay their interpretation of events and give their perspective on situations promotes awareness and provides opportunities for changing future responses. In order for adolescents to feel safe enough to engage in the process nurses need to demonstrate a respectful and accepting approach towards them. Successful and respectful validation of young people's thoughts and emotions enables them to identify the initial causes of their feelings, neutralize the associated emotions and help transfer them to remote memory once they have been dealt with. This process allows for further exploration of more appropriate responses and an improved ability to manage adversity.

Helping young people achieve mastery

The impact of the environment on the course of mental illness is well documented, particularly the relationship between nurse and patient and how this impacts on care (Lawson 1998; Yurkovich 1989; Geanellos 2002), yet the specific skills and functions of the nursing role are less clearly defined and often intuitively derived (Delaney 1992). Rowe (1988) suggests that knowledge of attachment theory is necessary as milieu treatment provides adolescents with a secure base that encourages them to explore pathways, to develop new relationships, to master new healthier patterns of behaviour, and to revise internal working models and develop more positive, facilitative ones. In performing these multi-dimensional roles nurses provide a continuous presence in the adolescent's environment, conveying a meaningful influence over the development of the ward cultures and norms. Nurses arbitrate between the physiological, psychological and social experience of the young person, utilizing actions, words and role modelling. Interventions are focused on both a group and an individual level, allowing the adolescents to learn both about their own needs and how to support others. Many nursing interactions will be associated with what may appear mundane everyday issues. However, it is the skilful observation and management of these everyday issues that establishes the supportive culture of the ward environment and supports the young people in learning how to manage their own issues and interpersonal relationships, thereby promoting psychological change and growth. One of the first tasks in the nurse/adolescent relationship is to develop a secure base for the adolescent, with the nurse acting as an attachment figure. Activities are organized so that the identified nurse is actively available for the young person, fostering the growth of a relationship and encouraging the young person's exploration and mastery of developmental tasks. Admission to an inpatient unit can often disrupt the adolescent's internal sense of self, causing validation of their internal sense of powerlessness and their image of themselves as 'bad' or 'defective'. Under these circumstances the adolescent may see the unit and staff as threatening or coercive, and this may cause them to become 'fixated' at a developmental phase that utilizes acting out behaviours that serve to distance the adolescent from the nurse and test the strength of the attachment relationship. Such behaviours are challenging for nurses as adolescents' sensitivities are often hidden beneath anger, sadness or confusion and may manifest as 'difficult' or withdrawn behaviours (Morse 1991). Developing an understanding of the specific clinical, developmental and relationship reasons as to why an adolescent may be reluctant to engage and participate is critical for nurses and essential for the adolescent. When nurses develop sensitivity to the adolescent's inner world they move beyond surface behaviours and respond to the person within (Delaney 1992). Nurses need to be able to decipher the adolescent's world view and adopt their frame of reference and internal working model, thereby allowing the adolescent to link past relationships with present behaviours and encourage the exploration of the pathway that their development has followed and to experiment with new, more competent behaviours and relationships. Nurses are less likely to react appropriately to adolescents' needs if they are unaware of the possible sources of tensions within the nurse/adolescent relationship.

'Limit setting' is identified as one of the principal goals of milieu treatment and is well practised in CAMHS nursing within inpatient settings. However this often adopts a classical behavioural therapy approach that may be in conflict with the attachment theory model of milieu therapy where limit setting occurs in the context of a relationship rather than in a vacuum. Therefore the quality of that relationship is most important for the effectiveness of the limit-setting intervention. This also applies to the development of self-regulation; Kopp's literature review (1982) emphasized the importance of the relationship to the caregiver in the development of self and internal controls.

The following case scenario provides an example of the application of the Gunderson Framework.

Box 10.1 Case scenario: the application of the Gunderson Framework

Two adolescents start to argue over the use of the TV in the evening after family visiting is over. One young person wants to use the Playstation, while the other wants to watch their favourite soap. The two boys initially start arguing about which of them gets priority over the remote. The other young people start taking an interest in the altercation. The argument becomes the focal point for the group and some of the observers start taking sides. The difference escalates to a point where tempers are rising with the potential for violence to develop.

- *Containment* – the situation was contained by the nurse stepping in and providing an authoritative stance. She reduced the rising tension by asking the observers to leave the scene, thereby also making the environment safer.
- *Structure* – the nurse intervened immediately, dealing with the two youngsters in a manner that was consistent with the unit rules and expectations. By also keeping calm the nurse was able to further reduce the rising tensions.
- *Support* – the nurse attended to the adolescents' verbal and non-verbal cues. By acknowledging their different perspectives but not taking sides she neutralized the situation further.
- *Involvement* – the two adolescents were made aware of how their initial behaviour impacted on the others within the community via the nurses facilitating the community meeting and helping the young people reflect on the process. Facilitation in this context is about enabling young people to express their feelings and views in socially acceptable ways. The involvement of all group members of the milieu ensured that everyone participated in the conflict resolution, enhancing group support and learning opportunities for all.
- *Validation* – the nurse facilitated listening not only to the two adolescents' perception of events but also the community's, indicating respect for the wider group and modelling effective communication.

Nursing in an acute inpatient adolescent unit

This section focuses on nursing in an acute inpatient unit. Oakham House is an eight-bedded unit, taking admissions from Leicester, Leicestershire and Rutland. The unit was originally opened in 1969 as an all-female unit operating Monday to Friday. It operated very much along the lines of a therapeutic community (as outlined above) for which there were strict admission criteria, or more importantly, exclusion criteria (anyone suffering from a psychotic illness was admitted to adult wards). The transition from a therapeutic community to an acute unit has been challenging and the nurses have had to develop their knowledge and skills accordingly.

Changes in clinical need combined with the publication of the *National Service Framework For Children* (DoH 2004) has resulted in an increasing expectation that inpatient units should be able to provide appropriate treatment on a 24-hour, seven days a week basis. Best practice advocates that adolescents under the age of 18 should not be admitted to adult wards unless that is deemed to be the most appropriate environment clinically. This has been made statutory in the Mental Health Act 2007. It will also become law, in April 2010, that should young people require admission to adult wards, it must be an age appropriate environment and they must have access to appropriate clinical staff and support services.

The skills referred to earlier in this chapter are important, as nurses are dealing with young people who are still developing and maturing. Nurses play a crucial role in maintaining this maturation process, despite the fact that the young person is experiencing a major illness which may detract attention away from achieving the goals of adolescence.

The nursing role on an acute inpatient unit

As a nurse working in an adolescent unit, you will have to be able to work effectively as a member of the nursing team and the wider multi-disciplinary team, while having the confidence and expert nursing knowledge to deliver care to the patients and families and contribute to the multi-disciplinary decision-making process.

Nurses often act as advocates for the adolescents on the ward. This important role may at times cause some differences within the team, and needs to be handled in an open, constructive and professional manner.

The nurses' behaviour and professional activities should, at all times, be guided by the Nursing and Midwifery Council's (NMC) code of practice (2008) and *The Ten Essential Shared Capabilities* (DoH 2007) listed below:

1 working in partnership;
2 respecting diversity;
3 practising ethically;
4 challenging inequality;
5 promoting recovery;
6 identifying people's needs and strengths;
7 providing service user centred care;
8 making a difference;
9 promoting safety and positive risk-taking;
10 personal development and learning.

Assessment on admission

The unit admits people between the ages of 12 and 18. They have to be suffering from, or suspected to be developing, a formal mental illness. It is sometimes difficult to ascertain whether a person is in a distressed state due to mental illness or social and family circumstances (admissions to alleviate social or family problems would be inappropriate). However, in an acute situation the young person may be admitted to clarify features of the presentation. As nurses will frequently have the greatest contact with patients, they are best placed to observe and assess them. They are also in an excellent position to provide a young person with support and act as advocate for them.

Nurses should complete the assessment in a systematic manner using the framework discussed in Chapter 5 and then carefully and accurately record and report their findings to the multi-disciplinary team in accordance with the NMC code of practice. Apart from nursing observations, it is also important to ask young people to self-assess. This will provide a useful view of their own feelings and can be cross-referenced with the nurse's observations.

As part of this assessment, or when a formulation has been made to start treatment, the nurses will be responsible for developing a care plan with the patient. The care plan should incorporate the following aspects:

- setting aims and objectives;
- identifying management techniques which are appropriate;
- assessing the skills of nursing team members.

Implementing the care plan

Once actioned, the care plans need to be regularly reviewed, updated and clearly documented. It is also good practice to have the plans signed by the patient and possibly their parents/carer and give them copies to keep.

Monitoring and evaluation is vital, so that once the aims of admission have been achieved, the patient can be discharged and returned to life in the community. Essentially, the care planning process was developed out of what we called the 'nursing process' in the 1980s, but the principles and structure are the same, involving assessing, planning, implementing and evaluation.

An intrinsic skill in nursing adolescents is good communication, both with colleagues and families, but the most vital aspect of communication is being able to establish a good rapport with the young people. Along with this aspect of the skills required, it is necessary for nurses to provide a sense of containment and safety to allow patients the security to work on their difficulties. Maintaining boundaries, for oneself and the young people, is important in order to retain a therapeutic relationship and an atmosphere that is conducive to treatment.

The skills mentioned above, to some degree, have to be part of a nurse's personality but are largely developed in a practical way from experience of doing the job. They will, however, be monitored and developed with the help of supervision, which should take place on a regular basis and at a minimum of one hour per month. Supervision can be individual or group and is used to explore feelings and thoughts about the work being undertaken, and also to develop skills and ensure that every nurse is practising safely and operating within their capabilities.

Specific aspects of inpatient nursing on an acute unit

Nurses are also responsible for maintaining a safe environment on the ward and delivering basic nursing care. With the opportunity within CAMHS to develop specialist therapeutic skills, the basic nursing requirements can easily be forgotten. Nurses need to attend to a young person's personal hygiene needs, ensure that they are taking adequate diet and fluids, monitor sleep and activity and record physical observations such as temperature, pulse, respiratory rates and blood pressure.

Management of actual or potential aggression (MAPA) is also an essential skill required on an inpatient unit. Situations can quickly develop where for the safety of the patient, or others, young people may need to be restrained. In most cases, however, skilled nurses are able to see situations developing and use their interpersonal skills to defuse the tension.

The management of risk is another central skill and activity in CAMHS. Our patients often present with some highly risky behaviours which have to be managed, while balancing this with remembering that one of the main tasks of adolescent development is to take risks. Using the care plan model, nurses need to assess the situation, taking all relevant factors into account and develop a risk management plan. The management of risk links clearly with our duty of care.

Due to the fact that many admissions involve severely ill young people, there is an increased need for the use of medication on inpatient units. Therefore inpatient nurses need a good working knowledge of pharmacology issues and an awareness of the policies relating to rapid tranquilization and relevant guidelines provided by the National Institute for Health and Clinical Excellence (NICE).

The care programme approach will be more commonly used in the inpatient setting, so nurses will have to be proficient in the use of the process and its documentation. This process, however, should be familiar to a profession which has a culture of good care planning and comprehensive risk assessments.

Using the Mental Health Act

A good working knowledge of the Mental Health Act 1983, amended in 2007, will also be required, as obviously not all patients will agree with the need for admission to hospital. The main changes that affect patients are as follows:

- under 18s must be treated in an environment suitable to their needs (this comes into force in April 2010); this applies to both detained and informal patients;
- duty on hospital managers to consult with appropriate clinician to establish what environment is appropriate for that young person;
- Trusts must tell courts and local authorities where CAMHS beds are located;
- patients under 18, who are not detained, will have a statutory right to advocacy for Section 58 treatments (i.e. electro-convulsive therapy, medication beyond three months);
- 16- and 17-year-olds, who have capacity, cannot have their wishes overruled by a person with parental responsibility.

Box 10.2 **Exercise**	• Having read about the two types of unit, from your own perspective what are the strengths and limitations of each type of approach?

Comparing and contrasting the two types of unit

Admissions are kept as short as possible on acute units as the main purpose is to undertake an assessment for any disorder or to stabilize the young person on treatment. Generally admissions last from overnight to a few weeks. This is often in contrast to therapeutic units. When Oakham House operated as a therapeutic community, admissions were planned for a minimum of six weeks but often lasted several months.

Acute units have the facility, and indeed are supported, to offer emergency admissions which can be vital to ensure the safety of acutely disturbed young people. Therapeutic communities tend to have little scope for unplanned admissions and often undertake a preadmission phase which can last several weeks. This means that the two types of unit are perhaps suited to addressing different problems. Acute units are staffed with professionals who are able to care for and manage acutely disturbed young people who may be very seriously mentally ill. Therapeutic communities on the other hand specialize in providing therapeutic support for relatively stable young people but provide only limited acute emergency care.

Box 10.3 shows the range of tasks undertaken by inpatient unit staff. Most tasks apply to both types of unit but the emphasis may be different. In acute units, the care is often started by inpatient unit staff and then transferred to community outpatient teams. This necessarily means that there has to be very good communication between inpatient unit staff and those working in the community.

Box 10.3 Typical tasks undertaken by inpatient unit staff (Royal College of Psychiatrists 1999)

- Care of basic needs: safety, nutrition, comfort and cleanliness.
- Maintenance of unit organization.
- Encouraging daily living skills.
- Maintaining healthy group dynamics among the young people through active early intervention and group work.
- Structured assessments including observations.

- Individual counselling of patients.
- Delivering specific psychological therapies such as cognitive behavioural therapy (CBT), anxiety management and family therapy.
- Delivering and monitoring medication.
- Taking part in team meetings or case conferences and care planning.
- Managing young people's contact with families, preparing for and debriefing after leave from the unit.
- Supporting parents/carers.
- Maintaining clear and effective communication between different staff.

Both types of unit will struggle to provide the level of care needed if the staff levels are kept to a minimum. Nurses are frequently placed under considerable stress as a result of inadequate provision of other appropriate staff (e.g. psychologists to provide CBT). Nurses also often have the responsibility for ensuring effective communication by the very fact that this is the professional group which is always present on the unit.

Staff dynamics in inpatient units can impact very significantly on the young people who can easily identify when staff are working together and when they are not. In the latter case, young people may play staff off against each other. It is an important factor that needs attention but may be less well addressed when units are understaffed, and staff feel unsupported. Effective leadership is a key factor in whether unit staff share a common purpose and one that is patient centred, or whether care is fragmented and incoherent.

Summary

Working in an inpatient unit is complex, particularly as in acute cases very seriously ill young people are often admitted. Additionally there is the intensity of the work involved as well as staff dynamics which can complicate the task further. As we know, admission to hospital is a useful and successful option for care but in the current changing climate of the National Health Service (NHS), inpatient units are equally under pressure to prove their effectiveness and evidence outcomes. In the context of this new business culture, it remains the nurse's own personal and professional responsibility to remain updated and open to new ways of working which are evidence based but still retain the caring component of the nursing role. The challenge for the profession is to retain the best of nursing while incorporating new developments into their roles.

References

Berliner, L. and Lipovsky, J. (1992) *Reframing Resistance As Avoidance*. San Diego, CA: Academic Press.
Butterworth, T. (1991) Generating research in mental health nursing, *International Journal of Nursing Studies*, 28(3): 237–46.
Delaney, K. (1992) Nursing in child psychiatric milieus, *Journal of Adolescents*, 5(1): 10–14.
DoH (Department of Health) (2004) *National Service Framework for Children, Young People and Maternity Services. Supporting Local Delivery*. London: DoH.
DoH (Department of Health) (2007) *The Ten Essential Shared Capabilities: A Framework for the Whole of the Mental Health Workforce*. London: DoH.
Geanellos, R. (2002) Transformative change of self: the unique focus of (adolescent) mental mealth nursing? *International Journal of Mental Health Nursing*, 11: 174–85.
Gunderson, J.G. (1978) Defining the therapeutic processes in psychiatric milieus, *Psychiatry*, 41: 327–35.

Killeen, M.R. (1990) Challenges and choices in child and adolescent mental health-psychiatric nursing, *Journal of Child and Adolescent Psychiatric and Mental Health Nursing*, 3(4): 113–19.

Kopp, C. (1982) Antecedents of self-regulation: a developmental perspective, *Developmental Psychology*, 18: 199–214.

Lawson, L. (1998) Milieu management of traumatised youngsters, *Journal of Child and Adolescent Psychiatric Nursing*, 11(3): 99–106.

Morse, J.M. (1991) Negotiating commitment and involvement in the nurse-patient relationship, *Journal of Advanced Nursing*, 16(4): 455–68.

NMC (Nursing and Midwifery Council) (2008) *The Code: Standards of Conduct, Performance and Ethics for Nurses and Midwives*, www.nmc-uk.org/aArticle.aspx?ArticleID=3057, accessed 20 August 2008.

Rowe, J. (1988) Attachment theory and the milieu treatment of children, *Journal of Child Psychiatric Nursing*, 1(2): 66–71.

Royal College of Psychiatrists (1999) *Guidance on the Staffing of Child and Adolescent Inpatient Psychiatry Units*. London: Royal College of Psychiatrists.

Yurkovich, E. (1989) Patient and nurse roles in the therapeutic community, *Perspectives in Psychiatric Care*, 25(3): 18–22.

Multi-agency working

Sarah Hogan, Nisha Dogra and Cath Kitchen

Key features
- The philosophy underpinning multi-agency working.
- The context for multi-agency working.
- Different types of multi-agency working examples from practice.
- The benefits and challenges for multi-agency working.
- Developing multi-agency working.

Introduction

In this chapter we begin by considering what multi-agency work is and the context of multi-agency working for specialist child and adolescent mental health services (CAMHS) nurses. The philosophy that underpins multi-agency working is discussed before different types of working are outlined. The potential benefits and challenges of such working are explored and these are used to suggest how good working practices can be set up. Examples are then provided of multi-agency working in practice.

The philosophy underpinning multi-agency working

Multi-agency working can be defined as a collaboration of work between different professional groups, agencies and sectors. It may involve two or more parties and may be informal, such as liaison and sharing information; or it may involve formal arrangements such as joint committees, planning, funding and strategies (DfES 2003). Multi-agency work may involve individuals from the same profession, coming from different organizational departments, or multi-disciplinary working, involving individuals with different professional backgrounds (Pettitt 2003). Wigfall and Moss (2001: 71) define multi-agency work as 'a range of different services, which have some overlapping or shared interests and objectives, brought together to work collaboratively towards some common purposes'. This definition is explicit that there needs to be a common goal which, as will be seen later, may be a crucial factor.

The *National Service Framework* (DoH 2004) clearly sets out a tiered service delivery model – that of universal, targeted and specialist support. It also states that it is for targeted support that multi-agency working is most effective; however, the justification for this claim is unclear. *Every Child Matters* (DfES 2003) advocates multi-agency working as an effective way of addressing the wide range of cross-cutting risk factors that contribute to poorer outcomes for children and young people. As a consequence, local authorities are currently reconfiguring their services to try to offer earlier, more coherent support in more convenient locations. This ties in with research by Tomlinson (2003), who, in her review, concludes that most good practice occurs at a local level rather than being a nationwide strategy, which seems to indicate that inter-agency working needs to be appropriate to context and developed in collaboration with all partners.

<table>
<tr><td>**Box 1.1**
Exercise</td><td>• What is your experience of working in multi-agency contexts?
• From your own experience, what did you identify as the potential benefits and challenges of such working?</td></tr>
</table>

The context for multi-agency working

The *National Service Framework for Children, Young People and Maternity Services* (DoH 2004) states that supporting children and young people with mental health problems should happen across all services, and is not the responsibility only of specialist child and adolescent mental health services (SCAMHS). There is an urgent need for nurses and other professionals to work across professional and organizational boundaries, and to function as collaborative, innovative and flexible practitioners.

Child and adolescent nurses in the UK work in a rapidly evolving policy and practice context, and are required to keep pace with strategic developments in education, welfare and youth justice. Innovations such as Sure Start, Connexions and the Children's Fund generate cross-cutting themes, and all require collaboration with mental health services. In schools, the Early Years Strategy, the Healthy Schools Initiative and Behaviour and Education Support Teams have shaped the work programme for school nurses. In welfare services, Quality Protects, Safeguarding Children and Therapeutic Fostering are all agendas to improve inclusiveness and the life chances of children looked after by the state. Each has mental health and resilience at its core. In youth justice, the Crime Reduction Strategy and the development of Youth Offending Teams both require close links with CAMHS.

CAMH nurses can direct the role of SCAMHS by working across inter-agency boundaries and developing networks and strategic links with policy-makers and children's planning forums including the Department of Health Nurse Advisors, the Children and Young People's Unit and Children's Taskforces (McDougall 2005).

The government, via *Every Child Matters* (DfES 2003), has proposed three broad models, multi-agency panels, multi-agency teams and integrated services, although it acknowledges that not all services fit the models exactly. We will look at each of these models in turn with examples of good practice.

Role of SCAMHS in multi-agency working

The *National Service Framework* (DoH 2004) clarifies that generic CAMHS should constitute a judicious combination of health, education, social services, housing, local amenities and the voluntary sector (Kurtz 2005). CAMHS is thus comprised of a variety of practitioners, including GPs, practice and school nurses, teachers and youth justice workers, and also mental health specialists who form part of specialist services but may also work at tier two (e.g. nurses working in specialist roles). The range of agencies involved makes the provision of CAMHS complex, and successful cross-agency working is vital. The Children Act 2004 has placed a duty on local authorities to make arrangements to initiate and promote cooperation between agencies, and a duty on key players to participate in this cooperation. With multi-disciplinary functioning as a key feature, integration of planning and commissioning of services by a single body with agreed strategies and a pooled budget should theoretically ensure effective cooperation between all the different services involved. It should also provide opportunities for children, young people and their families to participate (UEANCB 2005). However, the competing service priorities and financial restraints may mean that in practice service development is led by political priorities rather than children's needs. For example, social services often support the development of CAMHS that helps the children they share responsibility for, such as looked-after children. As they have less responsibility for children in general, the pressures that they are faced with may drive them towards a particular outcome. Within SCAMHS some cases will have a more obvious need for multi-agency working than others (e.g. when there are social or educational concerns). This is further illustrated later in the chapter. One of the most practical advantages of multi-agency working which includes the family is that there can be a single clear management plan that everyone is working towards. This can ensure that the family does not receive conflicting information from the different professionals involved in their care. It also affords the professionals some support and can ensure that they are not misinformed or misunderstand other partner roles. In practice, it has been most successful when there is mutual respect for each role and a clarity that each partner has more to gain than to lose by being involved in the work. Most importantly of all it meets the young person's needs. Once there has been a successful outcome, the next time it is easier to establish the work and vice versa. Salmon (2004) outlines the role of SCAMHS in multi-agency working. She also argues that much work needs to be undertaken on the language and definitions used between agencies before children's needs and the services they require can be developed.

Models for multi-agency working

Multi-agency panels

Practitioners on multi-agency panels remain employed and governed by their home agency. As the name implies, they meet as a panel on a regular basis to discuss children and young people with complex or additional needs who might benefit from a multi-agency approach to their support. As part of their work with the panel, the panel members or their home agency may carry out case work as part of a multi-agency plan.

Practice example

An example of this type of working arrangement is the Inter-agency Forum for School Non-attenders in Northamptonshire. Practitioners from CAMHS (psychiatrist and primary mental health worker), Connexions, the Pupil Referral Unit for pupils with medical needs, the behaviour support team, a mental health teacher, the children missing education team, education welfare services and a school nurse attend a panel once a month to discuss cases where children and young people are not attending school but who do not meet with admission criteria for any particular team. The cases are presented by different agencies, usually education welfare officers, and panel members are senior enough to be able to offer support from their own agency without consultation.

Multi-agency teams

A multi-agency team has a more formal configuration than a panel. In these teams, practitioners may be seconded or recruited to work full time in the team. Each team has an agreed leader and they work to a common purpose and goal, while maintaining links with their home agencies. These links may be through supervision and training or part-time work. These teams are therefore free to engage in work with more of the universal service and at a variety of levels (e.g. not

Table 11.1 Benefits and challenges of multi-agency panels

Benefits	Challenges
There are no recruitment or human resource issues as practitioners remain employed by a home agency while contributing to the multi-agency work	A lack of regular contact can make it hard to develop effective partnerships
Practitioners remain members of their home agency and access training and development opportunities through the home agency	Tendency for practitioners to identify with home agency rather than the multi-agency work
Practitioners have opportunities to work together and get experience of different working styles and remits	Practitioners may have no real resources identified for the multi-agency work
Where multi-agency panels are working effectively, the lead professional is given authority to carry out their role	Planning meetings can take up a considerable amount of time

Table 11.2 Perceived benefits and challenges of multi-agency teams

Benefits	Challenges
A good sense of team identity and co-working is at the heart of the team's approach	Recruitment
Communication is straightforward and joint training is easy to facilitate	Lack of time and resources identified to set up and develop such teams
Opportunities to carry out preventive and early intervention work in school and early years settings as well as small group and individual casework	Some teams can be 'virtual' teams and therefore have difficulty communicating, resulting in significant challenges

just with individual children and young people, but also with small groups, families and even whole-schools work).

Practice example

An example of this type of working is behaviour and education support teams (BESTs). These teams bring together a range of professionals working to support schools, families and children who are at risk of developing behavioural, emotional and/or attendance problems. The teams are made up of staff from education, social care, health and other services, the minimum number of members being four or five. The target for such teams was set by the Department for Education and Skills (DfES) and was to focus on identification, prevention and early intervention in order to promote emotional well-being, positive behaviour and school attendance.

An evaluation of the BEST teams was undertaken by Halsey *et al.* (2005) and identified a number of positive outcomes from working in these teams. They found that having a larger, more diverse range of professionals working in a team made referrals more streamlined and access more immediate. Professionals working in the teams felt that they had gained in terms of exchange of knowledge and expertise with other agencies but that sufficient time was needed for planning the provision and to ensure that the necessary infrastructure and resources were in place before the team became fully operational. As might have been anticipated, one of the early challenges encountered was the need for staff to adapt their practice from working individually as a specialist to working as a member of a multi-agency team.

Integrated services

Integrated services, as the name implies, are centres where a range of separate services share a common location and have a management structure that facilitates integrated working, including a commitment by partner agencies to fund and facilitate the service. Integrated services is a 'one stop shop' for the community with services working together, generally located in early years or school settings.

Practice example

Examples of integrated working can be found in Sure Start centres and 'extended schools'. The extended schools initiative was launched by the DfES in 2003. The original aim of them was to support at least one school in each local authority area to provide a comprehensive range of services, which would include access to health and adult learning as well as study support and child care from 8 a.m. to 6 p.m. Most of the first extended schools projects were based in disadvantaged areas. As might have been expected, these services were very diverse as schools charted the direction of the services in response to what they saw as local need. However, some common features were identified such as a focus on overcoming pupils' barriers to learning, a recognition that they were part of what were seen as family and community problems and that they were part of the additional provision to solve these. Additional staff were deployed in partnerships to deliver the provision and multiple funding streams were needed to support it (Cummings *et al.* 2007).

Multi-agency staff were not always based full-time in the schools, but services were offered in a more flexible way. Involving other professionals in discussions with the school-based inclusion team led to more effective working practices. This was important as there could not be a universal model, given the differing local contexts and needs. However, this can also be a cause of tension as the development of such a provision required that support be tailored to the school's working practices and priorities, while other external agencies and the local authority were seeking to provide area-wide provision. This is realistically a conflict between the extended schools being seen as the centre for the child, family and community provision and the schools being regarded as a contributor to wider area strategies.

Successful extended schools have developed partnerships with a range of statutory and voluntary agencies providing services to local children, families and communities, and these partnerships have taken time and trust to build up.

Table 11.3 Benefits and challenges of integrated services

Benefits	Challenges
Opportunity to address full range of issues relating to health in a non-stigmatizing universal setting	Requires rethinking early years services and their place in the community
Knock-on benefits for educational standards	How can partners be brought on board through 'collaborative leadership'?
Opportunities for joint training	Difficulties in developing a sense of identity or purpose
Shared base enhances communication between different services	Managing differential pay structures and working conditions

The current evidence base for multi-agency working

Multi-agency working has recently received a lot of attention because of its propagation by the UK government in health implementation strategies. The agenda has been pushed forward more on the basis of political ideology than a truly evidence-based approach. Several literature reviews on multi-agency working are available which deal with one specific sector or issue, but do not consider multi-agency working across a broad spectrum of activities. The potential outcomes from multi-agency working will now be explored.

Improved and more effective services

The most commonly identified benefits of multi-agency working were improved and more effective services and joint problem-solving. Lesser identified benefits were the ability to adopt a holistic approach, and increased understanding and trust between agencies (Atkinson *et al.* 2007). However, it is unclear how much of the evaluation work was truly independent.

Benefits for staff and services

The positive impact on professionals involved in multi-agency working was quite strong and well evidenced (Atkinson *et al.* 2002, 2007). The positive impact centred on the multi-agency activity being rewarding and stimulating, increased knowledge and understanding of other agencies, and improved relationships and communication between agencies.

Practitioners with backgrounds in single, traditional agencies reported high levels of satisfaction with multi-agency working, with feelings of liberation and broad-mindedness (Fitzgerald 2004). Schools delivering extended services reported opportunities for staff to work flexibly and access more career development opportunities, and experienced improvements in staff recruitment, retention and workload. School security and community partnerships were also enhanced (Pettitt 2003). The *On Track* evaluation identified positive impacts for the staff in the form of lesser replication of services, better links between the service providers, opportunities for professional development and career progression, more involvement in community development, and improved awareness of services and public perceptions of service providers (NfER 2004).

Improved outcomes for children and families

In the work reviewed by Atkinson *et al.* (2002, 2007) the impact on service users was not much documented and researched so it may be that the key purpose for multi-agency working was not actually met. While the reports on service users were comparatively few, the main impact appeared to be improved access to services through speedier and more appropriate referral and a greater focus on prevention and early intervention. More focused support was reported to improve the lives of service users. It is argued that joint work by multiple agencies resulted in the improved happiness, behaviour and well-being of children, better peer relationships and improved academic performance (Pettitt 2003). However, how such conclusions are drawn is often unclear. Sloper (2004) only found improved outcomes in one example. Most families and individuals with complex needs are required to maintain contact with multiple agencies and professionals. Most desire a single point of contact in the form of a single, trusted, named person to coordinate assessment, information-sharing and care pathways, to ensure quicker access to the right kind of support (Mukherjee and Sloper 1999). This can be achieved by appropriate understanding between the various agencies involved.

Factors influencing multi-agency working

Successful multi-agency working was dependent upon some important and crucial points including: the clarification of roles and responsibilities; securing of commitment at all levels; development of trust, mutual respect and understanding; effective communication and information-sharing; effective management and governance; and, lastly, securing adequate and sustained funding and adequate time allocation for the proposed work (Atkinson *et al.* 2001, 2002, 2007; Tomlinson 2003).

The potential challenges of multi-agency working are less often written about but usually are the opposite of those identified as crucial for success and include:

- different core functions, values, cultures, ethics and practice between different agencies that are not recognized, acknowledged or addressed;
- different service priorities and remits;
- lack of clarity with lines of authority and accountability;
- lack of ring-fenced resources;
- local history and tensions including previous history of agencies working together;
- conflicting and contradictory policy;
- lack of agreed purpose for each agency's involvement;
- differential power structures;
- multi-agency forums being used as a way of shifting resources onto another agency;
- when partners do not deliver as agreed;
- when the benefits are questionable.

Sloper (2004) has however argued that there is little evidence on the effectiveness of multi-agency working itself or on different models of such working in producing outcomes for children and families. She argues that the facilitators and barriers are now well established but that there is a need for methodologically sound research which investigates the outcomes of different models, including their cost effectiveness, and identifies the ways in which facilitating factors relate to outcomes.

Box 11.2 **Exercise**	• How does your own experience resonate with the evidence presented here? • What, if any, problems are there with the evidence that is given for multi-agency working?

Developing multi-agency working

Unfortunately, there is no precise formula for successful multi-agency working. It is complex as it involves different agencies, their procedures and protocols. It is challenging, as practitioners may be asked to 'step outside the box' and be more flexible. Most significantly, it is influenced by the individual personalities involved and the local context of the work. There is also some innocence in the benefits identified, in that sharing a base does not in itself bring about ease of communication or address the different perspectives that individuals bring. People do not suddenly start seeing benefits because a political directive tells them they should. It would not be unreasonable to assume that the same level of scrutiny be applied to the evidence being used to 'sell' multi-agency working as is used for other aspects of service planning and delivery.

Careful planning and negotiation is key, and shared goals and common targets are a good place to start. However, getting there can present a real challenge. Getting beyond what the group is about and what words can be used to talk about mental health are real challenges. The notion that stigma disappears if services are set in a universal setting is not borne out in practice, and the evidence in Chapter 1 shows that despite many interventions stigma remains a key issue.

A particular local need may be the reason for the instigation of a multi-agency partnership, which will provide the most obvious goal or target. Local data, combined with appropriate outcome measures, can then be used to indicate whether the project is having an impact and where improvements might need to be made. The multi-agency work should not be an end in itself, but should bring about benefits for children and their families that could not have otherwise been achieved by one agency working alone. The anticipated benefits should provide a clear vision which can then be translated into realistic goals, based in sound local knowledge of the needs of the target group and the support available to meet those needs. The goals may need to be revised as the project proceeds and in the light of experience. Governance arrangements need to be in place to ensure that appropriate accountability and oversight of the partnership agreements take place. Building on what is already in place is helpful and can help to facilitate communication through existing channels.

Box 11.3 Principles of good multi-agency working

- Clearly agreed and defined functions and goals.
- Tasks with agreed boundaries.
- Clear communication pathways.
- Clear understanding of each party's role and skills.

The setting of clear role definitions, possibly through a partnership agreement, is helpful in maximizing the contributions of each agency, avoids overlap and ensures that all agencies have equal contributions. However, bringing individuals from different professional backgrounds into a single team can be challenging for managers. Not only are there the different professionals cultures, but also questions about future career development, differences in pay and conditions, line management and joint training. However, multi-agency working should be seen as an important professional skill in itself. The meaning of this in practice may be difficult to define. Atkinson *et al.* (2002: vi) raise the idea of 'A new "hybrid" professional type, who has personal experience and knowledge of other agencies'. However, the value of multi-agency working may be lost as the expertise of each of the partners becomes diluted.

Partnership agreements

Partnership agreements are helpful in documenting the ground rules for working with different agencies in different contexts. This will help to ensure that the partnership has a firm foundation which will withstand any changes in personnel or other problems. Regular reviewing of the agreement ensures that these are 'living documents' and if they contain the identified goals and targets for the work, they serve as a useful reminder to agencies. Accurate and comprehensive information exchange is obviously an essential part of any multi-agency work. This requires an agreement on what information should be shared and, when dealing with specific cases, how this information should be exchanged and transferred to other agencies. The issue of accountability is also key. The idea that teams share responsibility may not be reflected when things go awry, as the recent coverage of Baby P will have demonstrated. Ayre (2008) comments that:

In principle *Every Child Matters* was the best thing to happen to children, in practice it created an 'audit culture' in the field of social care. It's now about ticking boxes and making sure that forms are filled out in time, being concerned with process and procedure instead of outcomes and objectives. Before *Every Child Matters* a nursery would telephone social workers to say that they were worried about a child, now they have to fill out a time-consuming common assessment framework form, so sometimes just don't bother ... Also as we move from child protection into safeguarding children I have seen cases in court where social workers' desire to work in partnership with parents can blunt their awareness to heavier issues that can result in a child's death.

This is perhaps a very vivid example of how the idea of effective multi-agency working in practice has very different outcomes than might be expected and of how practice can be very different from rhetoric.

Appropriate referral systems both into and out of multi-agency services ensure that these do not become a 'gap filler' for individual agencies. It is important that they deliver 'added value' and do not fulfil a function that is already being met by one of the home agencies. Exit strategies are useful to focus on the end point from early on in the planning process. Care should be taken, however, that the child and their family do not then become lost at the conclusion of the work.

In Box 11.4 we highlight an example of multi-agency working in practice through a clinical case.

Box 11.4 Case scenario

Hannah is 13 years old and was referred to SCAMHS by her GP with poor self-esteem, weight loss, low mood and superficial self-harm. Once Hannah had been assessed, it became clear that there were significant family issues and the relationship between Hannah and her mother was particularly fraught. Hannah's father had a better relationship with his daughter but found himself unable to manage the tensions between his wife and Hannah. Hannah was offered some individual work to help manage her behaviours concerning food (she did not meet the diagnostic criteria for any mental health disorder) and the family were also offered family therapy, which they refused. Hannah disengaged from the service by stating that the sessions made her feel worse. SCAMHS agreed with the family to keep the case open as they did not think things had been resolved. Several months later Hannah was referred through the on-call service, having taken an overdose. It emerged that she had been superficially cutting herself in response to arguments with her parents. The family stated they would like help but in family sessions neither Hannah not her parents engaged with the process. Over the next few months Hannah's self-harm escalated to such an extent that she had two admissions to the inpatient unit where she was quickly discharged as it became very evident that she did not have a mental disorder. The school nurse became involved in offering Hannah some support as she once again disengaged from CAMHS.

As Hannah's self-harm escalated, the family was referred to social services as the risk that Hannah presented related to her social context rather than a mental health disorder. Her parents also felt that the family was at breaking point and that they could no longer manage Hannah at home. A multi-agency meeting was convened. At the meeting, SCAMHS agreed to provide support for the school nurse who would continue to offer informal support as Hannah did not feel ready for any other work. Social services agreed to undertake an assessment of the family to look at the options of respite care and/or intense support within the family home.

In a case like Hannah's, the advantages of multi-agency working can be that there is a single management plan with each agency playing a clear part. This can prevent the family from presenting to each agency with conflicting pictures and blaming agencies for failing to make things better. In such situations, it is useful to identify the lead agency.

Multi-agency working is a key aspect of working with children and especially vulnerable young people (see Chapter 12). There have been some interesting service examples reported in the literature (Vostanis 2007).

Children and young people from vulnerable groups may not present with definable mental health problems but instead present with significant emotional and psychological distress that has a pervasive impact on their functioning (Minnis and Del Priore 2001; Hart and Luckock 2006). This can potentially lead to a misunderstanding between professionals in other agencies of what constitutes mental health and when a concern is underpinned by a mental health problem and who should take the lead. In the case scenario above social services had to be persuaded that the family context was the factor that maintained and escalated the self-harm risk. Unless that issue was addressed, Hannah would have been unable to utilize the other forms of support made available to her. However, it was important that SCAMHS remained involved until such a time that the risk was reduced and the family able to access support.

Summary

Multi-agency working has become a political imperative. There is limited evidence about whether the way that the government hoped it would work in practice has actually materialized. The programmes that are described as successes are often case studies and the generalizabilty to other contexts is unclear. Effective partnerships depend on mutual respect and some degree of shared values and/or purposes. This is a process that takes time and nurturing. It is arguable that the principles behind multi-agency working have merit when they are not about political or agency agendas, but when they are implemented in the best interests of young people.

References

Atkinson, M., Wilkin, A., Stott, A. and Kinder, K. (2001) *Multi-Agency Working: An Audit of Activity* (LGA Research Report 17). Slough: NfER.

Atkinson, M., Wilkin, A., Stott, A., Doherty, P. and Kinder, K. (2002) *Multi-Agency Working: a Detailed Study* (LGA Research Report 26). Slough: NfER.

Atkinson, M., Jones, M. and Lamont, E. (2007) *Multi-Agency Working and its Implications for Practice: A Review of the Literature.* Reading: CfBT.

Ayre, P. (2008) The audit culture feeds the climate of fear, blame and mistrust, www.guardian.co.uk/society/2008/nov/20/baby-p-child-protection, accessed 2 February 2009.

Cummings, C., Dyson, A., Muiji, D., Papps, I., Pearson, D., Raffo, C., Tiplady, L., Todd, L. and Crowther, D. (2007) *Evaluation of the Full Service Extended Schools Initiative: Final Report.* Slough: NfER.

DfES (Department for Education and Skills) (2003) *Every Child Matters: Change for Children.* London: DfES.

DoH (Department of Health) (2004) *National Service Framework for Children, Young People and Maternity Services: Supporting Local Delivery.* London: DoH.

Fitzgerald, M. (2004) Multi-agency working: literature review (unpublished).

Halsey, K., Gulliver, C., Johnson, A., Martin, K. and Kinder, K. (2005) *Evaluation of Behaviour and Education Support Teams*, Research Report RR706. Slough: NfER.

Hart, A. and Luckock, B. (2006) Core principles and therapeutic objectives for therapy with adoptive and permanent foster families, *Adoption and Fostering*, 30: 29–42.

Kurtz, Z. (2005) Assessing need, mapping services, and setting priorities, in R. Williams and M. Kerfoot (eds) *Child and Adolescent Mental Health Services: Strategy, Planning, Delivery, and Evaluation*. Oxford: Oxford University Press.

McDougall, T. (2005) Child and adolescent mental health services in the UK: nurse consultants, *Journal of Child and Adolescent Psychiatric Nursing*, 18(2): 79–83.

Minnis, H. and Del Priore, C. (2001) Mental health services for looked-after children: implications from two studies, *Adoption and Fostering*, 25: 27–38.

Mukherjee, B. and Sloper, P. (1999) *Unlocking Key Working: An Analysis of Keyworker Services for Families with Disabled Children*. Bristol: The Policy Press.

NfER (National Foundation for Educational Research) (2004) *Qualitative Study of the Early Impact of On Track*. Slough: NfER.

Pettitt, B. (2003) *Effective Joint Working Between Child and Adolescent Mental Health Services (CAMHS) and Schools*. Mental Health Foundation (DfES) Research Report RR 412. London: Mental Health Foundation.

Salmon, G. (2004) Multi-agency collaboration: the challenges for CAMHS, *Child and Adolescent Mental Health*, 9: 156–61.

Sloper, P. (2004) Facilitators and barriers for coordinated multi-agency services, *Child Care, Health and Development*, 30(6): 571–80.

Tomlinson, K. (2003) *Effective Interagency Working: A Review of the Literature and Examples from Practice*, LGA Research Report 40. Slough: NfER.

UEANCB (University of East Anglia and National Children's Bureau) (2005) *National Evaluation of Children's Trusts: Realising Children's Trust Arrangements. Phase I Report*. London: DfES/DoH.

Vostanis, P. (ed.) (2007) *Mental Health Interventions and Services for Vulnerable Children and Young People*. London: Jessica Kingsley.

Wigfall, V. and Moss, P. (2001) *More Than The Sum of its Parts? A Study of a Multi-agency Network*. London: National Children's Bureau.

Further reading

Donnelly, R.R. (2007) *Child and Adolescent Mental Health Services: Primary Mental Health Work*. Edinburgh: Scottish Executive.

RCN (Royal College of Nursing) (2007) *Lost in Transition: Moving Young People Between Child and Adult Health Services*. London: RCN.

12 Working with vulnerable children and young people

Viki Elliott and Panos Vostanis

Key features
- Who is vulnerable?
- Factors to consider when working with vulnerable groups.
- Challenges in working with vulnerable children and young people.

Introduction

This chapter begins by defining those young people who may belong to groups identified as vulnerable. The challenges for nurses and other clinicians of working with such people are discussed, as is the importance of staff ensuring that they have the opportunities to offload some of the pressures that may come with the role. Although it is difficult to determine the extent of children's vulnerability, some young population groups often stand out in their exposure to trauma, which consists of severe and ongoing adversities such as physical, sexual and/or emotional abuse and neglect, experience of domestic violence within the family and family conflict or breakdown (Vostanis 2004). These have a direct impact on their mental health and well-being, but also indirect effects through secondary difficulties – for example, offending, school exclusion or substance abuse, along with multiple changes in their life circumstances such as being placed in public care or becoming homeless. In this chapter we use adopted and looked-after children as an example to illustrate the specific issues that clinicians may need to consider when working with vulnerable groups. Multi-agency working, which is a key feature of working with vulnerable groups, is not covered in this chapter as the issues are addressed in Chapter 11. It is also well addressed in relation to vulnerable children in Vostanis (2007).

Who is vulnerable?

Vulnerable groups include children and young people who are:

- looked after either by foster families or by social service homes;
- children placed for adoption and adopted children;
- young offenders;
- homeless children;
- refugees and asylum seekers (who may be unaccompanied or with their families);
- from minority ethnic groups;
- considered to have a physical or learning disability.

Some young people will belong to several of these groups and it is unclear whether this has a cumulative impact on their mental health.

Evidence on the nature and interrelated features of mental health problems experienced by vulnerable children and young people will be considered in this chapter, followed by the implications for services and professionals involved, with particular reference to mental health nursing. There is good evidence that children from all categories identified as vulnerable are at increased risk of developing mental health problems (e.g. foster care, Meltzer *et al.* 2003; young offenders, Anderson *et al.* 2004). Children who belong to these groups often have strong environmental factors that are relevant in the development of mental health problems. For example, the reasons for family homelessness are diverse – predominantly domestic violence, relationship breakdown and neighbourhood harassment. A number of studies have found associated risks such as child protection, lack of social support, accidents and injuries, mental health problems among children and parents, and learning difficulties (Buckner *et al.* 1999; Webb *et al.* 2001).

Refugees and asylum seekers and some from minority ethnic groups, in addition to other factors, may experience social adjustment difficulties related to cultural, language and socio-economic factors. The experience of these groups both prior to, and following, arrival in the country of 'refuge' potentially increases their vulnerability to experiencing mental health problems. Many refugees and asylum seekers may have experienced the effects of war, social disruption and abuse.

The service context of meeting vulnerable children's and young people's mental health needs

Vulnerable children are less likely to exhibit defineable mental health problems, instead presenting with significant psychological and emotional distress that has a pervasive impact on their functioning, which may lead to misunderstanding between other agencies regarding what constitutes a mental health problem. Despite the well established level of vulnerable children's needs, emerging evidence suggests that these needs are not often adequately met. The underpinning reasons are fairly complex and relate to a mismatch between service systems and children's characteristics, rather than necessarily a lack of, or non-response, from services. Vulnerable children, almost by definition, usually have multiple needs that involve several agencies. Agency contacts may be initiated sequentially or in parallel, rather than in an integrated, more clinical and cost-effective way.

The referral criteria used by specialist child and adolescent mental health services (CAMHS) can cause tension between agencies, in particular for children with less severe mental health presentations, or with a broad spectrum of behaviours (within the remit of attachment or oppositional/conduct disorders) that cannot be addressed by a single agency or intervention (Vostanis *et al.* 2003). Other reasons include the lack of stability in the child's immediate care environment, moves between different areas (hence changes in schools and primary health care services that act as entry points to specialist provision) and social exclusion that can further disengage older adolescents from services and treatment. This pattern has been identified by studies with looked-after children (Vostanis *et al.* in press), young offenders (Kataoka *et al.* 2001), homeless families (Vostanis and Cumella 1999) and single homeless young people (Taylor *et al.* 2007b). These service gaps have been identified by recent policies in the UK, and have set the scene for the development of more appropriate services and interventions (DfES 2003; DoH 2004).

Engaging young people, families and their carers

When working with vulnerable children and young people several factors have an impact, consequently the process of engagement is likely to be relatively lengthy and ongoing and breaks are likely to occur in the process of the work. For children who have experienced abuse, neglect and trauma, entering into new relationships is likely to be challenging and frightening; as therapeutic work involves a significant focus on relationships, it is essential that we recognize the difficulties this presents for vulnerable children and young people. They are likely to have experienced adults as inconsistent, abusive, uncaring and not to be trusted (Hughes 2004). It is thus understandable that attempts to engage and offer intervention are met with covert or overt resistance and avoidance (Howe and Fearnley 2003). This may lead to a conflict in organizational response, with different teams interpreting and responding differently to, for example, guidance on non-attendance (Edwards 2007).

Children may have been misled regarding the reasons for and possible outcome of attendance, further disempowering the young person and potentially mirroring previous experiences. Past contact with professionals and the consequent perception of this seems to significantly increase children's anxiety – for example, many fostered or adopted children seen in clinical practice are concerned that attendance is linked with removal from their foster or adoptive family. It appears to be beneficial to voice the possible range of worries that a child may have at the initial meeting to alleviate some of these worries. Clinical experience suggests that young people do not verbalize these concerns, but readily acknowledge them when labelled by the therapist.

Who to focus on?

On occasions it may be more appropriate to work exclusively with significant adults rather than directly with the young person. Such work is likely to involve assisting these adults to increase their understanding of the impact of the abuse, neglect, trauma and inconsistent care the young person has experienced, helping them to better understand the underlying emotions rather than focusing on the expressed behaviour. As a result carers are more able to reframe the issues and difficulties, thus enabling a shift in their views of their children to seeing them as traumatized, distressed, anxious and confused, as opposed to naughty and oppositional.

Hierarchy of needs

It is also helpful for adults to have an understanding of the hierarchy of the needs of vulnerable children to reduce the emphasis that may be placed on therapeutic intervention as opposed to their broader needs, and the significance of adapting environmental and social factors to meet those needs (Dent and Golding 2006). The need for a child to feel emotionally, physically and psychologically safe cannot be underestimated, although this can present one of the greatest demands on parents and professionals working with children whose experiences have continuously reinforced a lack of containment and safety. The benefits of therapeutic intervention require careful communication, to clarify the rationale and objectives of an approach, and the significant role of parents and carers within the therapeutic relationship.

Box 12.1 Case scenario

Peter, aged 8, was referred to CAMHS. He had a history of chronic sexual, emotional and physical abuse and neglect. He was adopted at age 4 along with his younger sisters, who had very different experiences than Peter. Peter was presenting with extreme anger and aggression, oppositional behaviour, was taking things from the family home, including food, and rejected any attempts by his adoptive parents to be close. Consequently, they had become increasingly frustrated and had begun to distance themselves from Peter physically and psychologically to protect themselves from the emotions generated by his behaviour. Peter met with a CAMHS nurse but it was clear that he was not currently able to engage in therapeutic work. Therefore, the clinician worked with the parents to assist them to develop and enhance their understanding of the impact of Peter's traumatic experiences, the rationale for the presenting behaviours and potential strategies to utilize in parenting Peter, while also considering their own emotional response and factors that had contributed to this. They engaged well in the work after an initial period of uncertainty, querying the clinician would work with them when it was 'Peter with the problem'. Through an increased understanding, the parents were able to reframe Peter's behaviour, putting this in context and consequently responding to his emotional needs rather than his presenting behaviour.

By its very nature, parenting work is wide ranging, with professionals in different agencies varying in their interpretation of the indications, framework and objectives of such work, and who should be providing such work can present significant challenges (Street and Davies 2002).

Addressing narratives and expectations

Narrative and expectations are important to consider in all children. However, when working with adopted, looked-after children and refugees there may be a temptation for parents, carers and other agencies to focus exclusively on historical issues, thinking about the experiences of neglect, abuse and trauma and their impact. Although these are obviously highly significant, the importance of considering current and future context should not be underestimated. Issues that arise in clinical practice would indicate a potential to place sole responsibility for the presenting difficulties on the birth family or individual child. For example, adoptive parents and carers often discuss the inevitability of their child being volatile and angry due to their genetic make-up and the history of anger and aggression in the birth family. As such, young people may find themselves in situations that become self-fulfilling prophecies due to their perception of themselves as 'bad', and the parental script that they have a predisposition towards anger and aggression. This can lead to distancing by both parties, thus further reinforcing the attachment difficulties and the child's negative blueprints.

Diagnosing children and young people with attachment disorders or attachment difficulties presents a further dilemma. While providing a label can increase the understanding of the issues and needs presented by a young person, attachment difficulties are not a rigid or fixed phenomena. Parents and professionals can sometimes attribute these difficulties as intrinsic to the child, consequently shifting the responsibility from them to support the child to enable progress, or reinforcing the belief that change is not possible, or that the child requires therapy in order to be 'fixed' (Street and Davies 2002). This can further impact on considering issues in the 'here and now' such as dynamics in a foster or adoptive family. Therapeutic work should therefore assist carers and professionals to move away from perceiving attachment as internal to the child to viewing this in the context of a relationship, i.e. a two-way process and shared responsibility (Minnis and Del Priore 2001).

Supporting children

Supporting children to develop a coherent narrative through life story work may be undertaken prior to commencing therapy or alongside therapy. Clinical practice suggests that young people often lack an age appropriate or realistic understanding of their life story. This not only exacerbates feelings of confusion about their experiences but also has an additional impact on their ability to integrate within the adoptive family, foster care placement or residential home. Therapeutic work could consider the process of the child's life story while the social worker provides a factual account of their experiences (Edwards 2007). Alongside this, parents and carers need to be assisted to support the child physically, emotionally and psychologically. They need to be prepared to contain the different and strong feelings that are likely to be evoked, such as sadness, anger, confusion, distress and relief, while being aware of their own emotional response. In doing so, they will give a powerful message to the child that the adults in their life can now manage the details of their life story, and can support them in processing their experiences of loss and grief while assisting them to integrate into their new family. Children can thus develop a 'narrative about self that is added to and embellished as they grow and understand at an increasingly mature level' (Golding 2008: 65).

Working individually with children and young people

Considering the appropriateness or timing of undertaking individual work with young people can present a further challenge, due to the potential risk of pathologizing and reinforcing the perception that the sole responsibility for change lies with the child.

There would seem to be ongoing debate and discussion about the need for a secure base prior to commencing therapeutic work and the timing of therapeutic interventions with children and young people. The need for children to feel safe and secure, contained, able to elicit care and comfort, and have their needs met at some level, and as such be able to undertake therapeutic work, may initially involve working with the parents or carers to assist and support them in further developing their relationships. However, this may be difficult to achieve without engaging with the child to some extent. Transitional issues and time within a placement or family need to be taken into account. However, professionals may be faced with the dilemma of potential family or placement breakdown if therapeutic work is not undertaken at some level, while considering the possible consequences of this. For example, the potential for challenging behaviour to escalate, and the inability of the young person to be contained, adding further pressure to an already unstable system. It may, therefore, be appropriate to consider issues in the here and now, permitting the child an opportunity to deal with their current anxieties and thereby providing a positive experience that will enable the child to access further therapeutic intervention if required in the future (Lanyado 2003).

Involving carers

It is well recognized that the involvement of parents and carers is fundamental for any work with vulnerable children and young people to be successful. This may take a variety of forms such as direct intervention with the child and their parents or carers, utilizing techniques suggested by Hughes (2004) and Jernberg and Booth (2001). These approaches would seem to further enhance understanding of the reasons for the young person's attachment and presenting difficulties and promote parental and carer involvement.

It may be appropriate that work is initially undertaken exclusively with parents to enable them to increase their understanding of the presenting difficulties, the impact of the child's experiences prior to leaving their birth family, the rationale for the current behaviour, strategies to utilize in parenting children with such needs, and their fundamental role in supporting the child to make progress, as well as providing support to enable them to tolerate the emotional and behavioural issues that might occur during the process of therapy (Allen and Vostanis 2005). This presents a further dilemma when contemplating the timing of work and with whom this should be undertaken. Anecdotal and clinical experience indicates that if parents and carers do not engage in therapeutic work, young people do not seem to make substantial progress or are prone to relapse. This is further exacerbated if parents have unresolved issues that they are unable or unwilling to explore.

Working with families and systems

Certainly when working with looked-after and adopted children a number of issues and dynamics arise that impact on the presenting difficulties, the care package and the progress made. The presenting needs of the child now in the adopting parents' care can trigger a number of feelings and responses that are then played out in the relationships within the family. The combination of the needs of both children and parents can have a significant impact on interactions, often observed as a 'push-pull' dynamic where there seems to be both a desire for, but fear of, a developing relationship. This may be further compounded by children re-enacting trauma, which is likely to be misinterpreted by parents and adds a further dynamic to an already fragile relationship. As such, parents and children may physically and/or psychologically reject each other (Hodges *et al.* 2003), consequently reinforcing the child's negative internal working models and potentially escalating challenging behaviours, resulting in a destructive and ongoing cycle that may ultimately lead to the family breaking down (Delaney 1998).

Vulnerable children and young people require parenting that replicates positive parent-child interactions, which need to be sensitive, responsive, empathic and attuned. Due to the strategies that have been developed by children to survive early experiences of abuse, neglect and trauma, parenting has to be sensitive and responsive to the expressed and hidden emotional needs (Golding 2008), thereby assisting them to rework experiences missed out on as a result of early life events. Hughes (2006) suggests that adults can remain emotionally engaged with vulnerable children and young people by enabling carers to become attuned to their child through a stance of playfulness, acceptance, curiosity and empathy, thereby assisting young people to feel connected, understood and validated (Golding 2008). It is hoped that having the experience of safe, empathic, reliable parenting will allow children to replace old mental representations of carers as dangerous and unreliable with more secure models of caregiving at times of need (Howe 2006). This will involve assisting parents and carers to improve children's emotional communication and regulation through labelling, and co-regulation of emotions. To do this, parents and carers also need to be aware of the importance of taking care of themselves and assisted to reintroduce fun and enjoyment into the family home.

The nursing role

Considering the role of the nurse in supporting parents and carers to parent their children therapeutically can further compound the dilemma of the timing of this intervention and who should undertake it. Whether this intervention is more successful when facilitated as part of a group also requires consideration. Clinical experience would indicate that a group-based intervention for adoptive parents appears to have better outcomes than when this work is undertaken individually. This links with opportunities for peer support and the value of the participants having a shared understanding of their experiences prior to and post adoption. Alongside this is the opportunity to share skills and strategies (Allen 2007; Niccols 2008).

To enable parents to undertake therapeutic parenting requires a degree of understanding on their part of traditional parenting techniques and strategies, along with the ability to empathize, nurture, reflect and acknowledge personal issues and emotional responses. Due to the nature of the child's difficulties and experiences there is likely to be disparity in their chronological and emotional development. A combination of this, the range of needs and presenting issues, and the different levels and stages of attachments in relationships, indicates that a mix of therapeutic and more traditional parenting is likely to be required to meet the needs of the child. Parents and carers may require additional support, advice and education to facilitate this. Consultation with other agencies may be the most appropriate intervention at such times. It is well recognized that consultation work has a central place in work with adoptive and foster families (Hart and Luckock 2006).

Parents, children and professionals may be constantly striving to achieve at an unrealistic level in terms of their own capacity or their child's ability, thereby further compounding a sense of disappointment and failure, leading to them further distancing themselves psychologically, emotionally or physically in order to protect against these emotions (Howe and Fearnley 2003). Issues from their own experience of being parented may be triggered leading to different dynamics in the parent, child and couple relationship (Hudson 2006). Parents who find themselves struggling to manage the many varied and complex needs presented by their children can begin to question their own abilities to parent.

The combination of these factors can lead to a fear of being judged, and consequently services and assistance may not be sought until the family is at crisis point and at potential risk of breaking down (Harris 2004). This would seem to be shifting gradually with the improvements in multi-agency training. However, it remains an issue for families who adopted some time ago.

The importance of considering the adults' own attachment style raises further issues regarding the timing and nature of interventions. Kaniuk *et al.* (2004) found that adopters with unresolved attachment issues were unable to focus on their child's needs adequately and often felt hurt and rejected by the challenging behaviours presented. Although most families did not break down, these children failed to progress in terms of developing more secure attachments and remained unable to manage relationships at home and school.

Challenges in working with vulnerable children and young people

The complex and interrelated needs of vulnerable children, young people and their carers, as well as issues arising from multiple agency involvement, can present a challenge when considering service design and delivery, as well as who is best placed to provide the service and the ways in which this may be achieved – for example, via generic or dedicated specialist teams (Minnis and Del Priore 2001). Specialist posts allow individual practitioners to develop and enhance the skills and knowledge base for this client group. The flexibility of nursing is particularly suited to the service needs of this young population, and nurses can play a central role in developing a coherent understanding and conceptual framework of appropriate services for the children and the systems around them: 'complex family and community contexts often confound traditional therapeutic methods, and organisational contexts are not always set up to deal effectively with them' (Hart and Luckock 2006: 31).

Specialist posts

Specialist posts can also remove dilemmas associated with access to services that may otherwise be bound by rigid criteria that prevent access for vulnerable groups, thereby minimizing the potential for conflict with existing practice and prioritization structures. However, one also needs to consider the risk of losing core/generic skills and experience of working with more definable mental health problems. This may occasionally lead to conflict within the organization, whereby children and young people do not fit specific diagnostic criteria and the work is more difficult to define in terms of duration and possible outcomes of intervention. Teams working with vulnerable children fit within the objectives for early intervention and prevention as identified in the *National Service Framework for Children, Young People and Maternity Services* (DoH 2004), but may be less compatible with new commissioning arrangements and 'payment by results', and this needs to be taken into consideration in strategic and operational planning.

Considering at what point CAMH nurses should begin and end their role presents an ongoing dilemma. It is often appropriate to offer inter-agency training and consultation to professionals, foster carers and adoptive parents, alongside any work that is being undertaken by CAMHS. This is a significant component of their role, but also one that can generate high levels of inter-agency conflict, with different professionals assuming the other is responsible for undertaking this work.

Funding issues

These challenges can be compounded by the funding arrangements that accompany designated posts in specialist teams, whereby the funding may have delineated a specific and occasionally inflexible remit. Other organizations may thus assume a degree of ownership of the posts, which may be influenced by their organizational pressures and priorities. In turn, this could lead to conflict regarding the nature, role and responsibilities of a particular post and the ways in which services should be designed and delivered. Joint planning and agreement are, therefore, essential before such posts are set up and processed.

Emotional impact

The emotional impact of the work is high, and there is potential for clinicians to burn out. Consideration needs to be given to where post-holders will be based and who will manage them. As they are often isolated roles, clinicians may struggle to maintain contact with the wider nursing team and may feel disconnected from it due to the different nature of their work. Professional isolation may potentially affect their working practices and personal stress levels (Taylor *et al.* 2007a).

Therapists undertaking work with clients with traumatic histories may find themselves overwhelmed by the nature, intensity and degree of the issues identified and reported (Turner 2000). They may feel de-skilled, or at risk of secondary traumatization. There may also be a desire to rescue the client, with workers feeling disempowered by the systems around them and their clients. The pace of work and path of progress with vulnerable children fluctuates and is often very slow. These feelings may mirror the experiences of the client group (young people, families and other professionals) and lead to parallel processes within the therapeutic work. Individual and peer supervision is a crucial mechanism to enable these issues to be considered and explored. Due to the specialist nature of the work there may be a need for discipline-specific or management supervision to be undertaken along with clinical supervision.

Vulnerable children and young people present with many and varied needs, and have multiple and recurrent contacts within the health and welfare systems. This highlights the need for inter-agency collaboration and cooperation between the agencies involved. Due to these complexities and multi-faceted issues, it is likely that children and young people will complete cycles of interventions that result in some level of improvement rather than a 'cure'. It may thus be helpful to anticipate that they may return for further therapeutic work in the future, as they go through different transitional phases and experiences that are likely to trigger further issues that may benefit from additional therapeutic interventions. It is important that this is acknowledged and not seen as failure on the part of the child or the therapy. Services that can offer continuity of care, clear care pathways and flexible re-referral criteria when difficulties re-emerge are, therefore, particularly valuable (Hart and Luckock 2006).

Summary

In this chapter we have identified vulnerable groups. We have used the needs of looked-after and adopted children as an example to illustrate the potential complexity of working with them. We have examined the challenges of working with such groups and how some of these challenges might be met. Throughout the chapter we have demonstrated that adults and agencies need to understand themselves and the different roles they may play in supporting the needs of such children. The need for staff to be aware of the impact of such work on themselves has also been highlighted.

References

Allen, J. (2007) Interventions for foster carers and adoptive parents of children who have experienced abuse and trauma, in P. Vostanis (ed.) *Mental Health Interventions and Services for Vulnerable Children and Young People*. London: Jessica Kingsley.

Allen, J. and Vostanis, P. (2005) The impact of abuse and trauma on the developing child: an evaluation of a training programme for foster carers and supervising social workers, *Adoption and Fostering*, 29: 68–81.

Anderson, L., Vostanis, P. and Spencer, N. (2004) Health needs of young offenders, *Journal of Child Health Care*, 8: 149–64.

Buckner, J., Bassuk, E., Weinreb, L. and Brooks, M. (1999) Homelessness and its relation to the mental health and behaviour of low-income school-age children, *Developmental Psychology*, 35: 246–57.

Delaney, R. (1998) *Fostering Changes: Treating Attachment-Disordered Foster Children*. Oklahoma City, OK: Wood & Barnes Publishing.

Dent, H. and Golding, K. (2006) Engaging the network: consultation for looked after and adopted children, in K. Golding, H. Dent, R. Nissim and L. Stott (eds) *Thinking Psychologically About Children who Are Looked After and Adopted: Space for Reflection*. Chichester: John Wiley.

DfES (Department for Education and Skills) (2003) *Every Child Matters: Change for Children*. London: The Stationery Office.

DoH (Department of Health) (2004) *National Service Framework for Children, Young People and Maternity Services: Child and Adolescent Mental Health*. London: DoH.

Edwards, V. (2007) Therapeutic issues in working individually with vulnerable children and young people, in P. Vostanis (ed.) *Mental Health Interventions and Services for Vulnerable Children and Young People*. London: Jessica Kingsley.

Golding, K. (2008) *Nurturing Attachments in Supporting Children who are Fostered or Adopted*. London: Jessica Kingsley.

Harris, P. (2004) Users' views and experiences of post-adoption services: a study of a regional post adoption agency, *Adoption and Fostering*, 28: 50–60.

Hart, A. and Luckock, B. (2006) Core principles and therapeutic objectives for therapy with adoptive and permanent foster families, *Adoption and Fostering*, 30: 29–42.

Hodges, J., Steele, M., Hillman, S., Henderson, K. and Kaniuk, J. (2003) Changes in attachment representations over the first year of adoptive placement: narratives of maltreated children, *Clinical Child Psychiatry and Psychology*, 8: 351–67.

Howe, D. (2006) Developmental and attachment psychotherapy with fostered and adopted children, *Child and Adolescent Mental Health*, 11: 128–34.

Howe, D. and Fearnley, S. (2003) Disorders of attachment in adopted and fostered children: recognition and treatment, *Clinical Child Psychology and Psychiatry*, 8: 369–87.

Hudson, J. (2006) Being adopted: psychological services for adopting families, in K. Golding, H. Dent, R. Nissim and L. Stott (eds) *Thinking Psychologically about Children who are Looked After and Adopted*. Chichester: John Wiley.

Hughes, D. (2004) An attachment-based treatment of maltreated children and young people, *Attachment and Human Development*, 6: 263–78.

Hughes, D. (2006) *Building the Bonds of Attachment: Awakening Love in Deeply Troubled Children*, 2nd edn. New York: Guilford Press.

Jernberg, A. and Booth, P. (2001) *Theraplay: Helping Parents and Children Build Better Relationships through Attachment-based Play*. San Francisco: Jossey-Bass.

Kaniuk, J., Steele, M. and Hodges, J. (2004) Report on a longitudinal research project, exploring the development of attachments between older, hard-to-place children and their adopters over the first two years of placement, *Adoption and Fostering*, 28: 61–7.

Kataoka, S., Zima, B., Dupre, D., Moreno, K., Yang, Z. and McCracken, J. (2001) Mental health problems and service use among female juvenile offenders: their relationship to criminal history, *Journal of the American Academy of Child and Adolescent Psychiatry*, 40: 549–555.

Lanyado, M. (2003) The emotional tasks of moving from fostering to adoption: transitions, attachment, separation and loss, *Clinical Child Psychology and Psychiatry*, 8: 337–49.

Meltzer, H., Gatward, R., Corbin, T., Goodman, R. and Ford, T. (2003) *The Mental Health of Young People Looked after by Local Authorities in England*. London: HMSO.

Minnis, H. and Del Priore, C. (2001) Mental health services for looked after children: implications from two studies, *Adoption and Fostering*, 25: 27–38.

Niccols, A. (2008) 'Right from the start': randomized trial comparing an attachment group intervention to supportive home visiting, *Journal of Child Psychology and Psychiatry*, 49: 754–64.

Street, E. and Davies, M. (2002) Constructing mental health services for looked after children, *Adoption and Fostering*, 26: 65–75.

Taylor, H., Stuttaford, M. and Vostanis, P. (2007a) Organisational issues facing a voluntary sector mental health service for homeless young people, *Journal of Integrated Care*, 15: 37–46.

Taylor, H., Stuttaford, M., Broad, B. and Vostanis, P. (2007b) Listening to service users: young homeless people's experiences of a new mental health service, *Journal of Child Health Care*: 11, 221–30.

Turner, S. (2000) Therapeutic approaches with survivors of torture, in J. Kareem and R. Littlewood (eds) *Intercultural Therapy*, 2nd edn. Oxford: Blackwell.

Vostanis, P. (2004) Impact, psychological sequalae and management of trauma affecting children, *Current Opinion in Psychiatry*, 17: 269–73.

Vostanis, P. (ed.) (2007) *Mental Health Interventions and Services for Vulnerable Children and Young People*. London: Jessica Kingsley.

Vostanis, P. and Cumella, S. (eds) (1999) *Homeless Children: Problems and Needs*. London: Jessica Kingsley.

Vostanis, P., Meltzer, H., Goodman, R. and Ford, T. (2003) Service utilisation by children with conduct disorders: findings from the GB national study, *European Child and Adolescent Psychiatry*, 12: 231–8.

Vostanis, P., Bassi, G., Meltzer, H., Ford, T. and Goodman, R. (in press) Service use by looked after children with behavioural problems: findings from the England survey, *Adoption and Fostering*.

Webb, E., Shankleman, J., Evans, M. and Brooks, R. (2001) The health of children in refuges for women victims of domestic violence, *British Medical Journal*, 323: 210–13.

13 Clinical governance, audit and supervision

Nisha Dogra and Dee Davies

Key features	• What is clinical governance?
	• Principles of effective clinical governance and applicability to child and adolescent mental health services (CAMHS).
	• What is audit?
	• Why audit?
	• How to audit.
	• The differences between audit and research.
	• What is supervision and how does it work?
	• Different models and types of supervision.

Introduction

In this chapter we cover clinical governance, clinical audit and supervision. Each of these roles is a major component for clinicians in terms of planning, managing and delivering effective clinical care. We begin by defining clinical governance and providing a brief history to give some context. Key themes for effective clinical governance are outlined as are the limitations of putting policy into practice. We then define audit and justify its importance to clinicians. The steps of an audit project are described and an example of an audit project undertaken within a CAMHS services is used to illustrate each step. The difference between audit and research is discussed before we move on to consider what supervision is and summarize the key points in two widely used models. Different types of supervision are reviewed before the effectiveness of supervision is discussed.

Clinical governance

The most widely used definition is that clinical governance is:

a system through which all NHS organisations are accountable for continually improving the quality of their services and safeguarding high standards of care by creating an environment in which excellence in clinical care will flourish.

(NHS Executive 1997 cited in Scally and Donaldson 1998: 61)

Clinical governance is a framework that overarches already existing mechanisms in place to improve health care, for example clinical audit, national guidelines, risk management and continuing professional development (CPD) (Scally and Donaldson 1998). The 'new' framework was provided with some resources and a number of policies. However, it is perhaps unsurprising that such a broad statement has led to widely varying interpretations. The impression given by such a statement is that we already know the factors that lead to 'an environment in which . . . care will flourish' when this is far from the case in practice.

Scally and Donaldson outline the origins of clinical governance. It was in many ways a political response to address concerns following several inquiries into serious National Health Service (NHS) shortcomings. Failures in breast and cervical screening programmes had also led to public confidence concerns about the NHS. Clinical governance was supposedly designed to consolidate, codify and universalize fragmented policies. A key aim was that through a framework (that was not specifically defined) some vehicle would become available which would continually improve the quality of patient care and develop NHS capacity.

Key principles for clinical governance from nursing frameworks

The Royal College of Nursing (RCN 2003) developed a number of key principles which underpin the implementation of clinical governance from a nursing framework, although mental health nursing was not specifically identified. The principles reflect key policy drivers at the time but other reasons or justifications are not given. The framework is outlined below and clinical examples given to illustrate the potential realization of policy into practice. The principles are as follows.

- *Clinical governance must focus on improving the quality of patient care.* In practice, clinical governance must be used to make and be shown to be making specific improvements to patient care (e.g. CPD is linked to improving the delivery of care).
- *The principles and framework apply irrespective of the context in which health care is delivered.* This means that clinical governance frameworks are applicable in inpatient and outpatient care and also when work is undertaken with other agencies.
- *Clinical governance needs 'true' partnerships between all stakeholders including patients.* The realization of this is difficult as it involves more resources, including time, than clinicians often have available. Patients still tend to be represented in a tokenistic way.
- *Clinical governance has public and patient involvement as an 'essential' requirement.* Again this appears to be stating a policy position rather than reflecting on how it applies in practice.
- *Clinical governance requires nurses to play a key role.* While this is a laudable principle, attention needs to be given to providing some detail as to how nurses can be involved. This is especially relevant in CAMHS when the nursing group may as a whole be smaller than in other areas. Poor resourcing of CAMHS may also mean that nurses have little protected time for such activity.
- *Clinical governance needs to create a culture which 'celebrates success and learns from mistakes'.*
- *Clinical governance applies to all health care staff.*
- *Clinical governance does not replace but complements individual clinical judgement or professional self-regulation.*

In *Clinical Governance: An RCN Resource Guide*, the RCN (2003) identifies the following themes as key for nurses:

- building blocks (including consultation and patient involvement, leadership, planning of services, performance reviews and health community partnerships);
- supporting nurses in the workplace through staff management, CPD and team working;
- quality improvement in action (including risk management, incident reporting, complaints, research and effectiveness and audit);

- placing the patient at the heart of health care, including planning and organization of care and environment of care.

All these themes assist and inform nurses when undertaking their professional roles. The guide, as it claims, is a resource and it usefully fills that role but it is perhaps rather accepting of the political rhetoric without appearing to question how improvements will be made.

The impact of clinical governance

Thomas (2002) raised the question as to whether there was any evidence to support the use of clinical governance to improve the quality of patient care. He also questioned whether clinical governance was based in any theoretical or intellectual context or whether it was merely political ideology.

It has been argued that clinical governance was as much about changing the culture of organizations as it was about emphasizing the principles behind the policy. The logic is that 'good' organizations are culturally different from those that are not good. However, what is considered a 'good' organization depends on many factors including political ideology and personal values (Balogun and Hope-Hailey 2004). The clinical governance framework is now widely used and usually referred to as accepted practice. However, it is unclear as to whether the concept is really understood or not, and whether any change has been made because of the framework.

Thomas's (2002) criticisms also reflect our personal experience of working within CAMHS. However, we would argue that although work has to date not shown the concept of clinical governance to have in itself led to any real improvement, that does not reduce the potential for change to be achieved. Scally and Donaldson (1998: 365) concluded that 'clinical governance is a big idea that has shown it can inspire and enthuse' and that many factors needed to come together to transform the concept into reality. Perhaps what is needed now is to review the potential benefits of clinical governance to CAMHS. It is unlikely that individual clinicians can change systems, however, every one of us can take responsibility for considering the issue of quality.

Box 13.1 **Exercise**	• Can you identify the clinical governance framework within your organization? • Who has lead responsibility for clinical governance? • Is there evidence that the framework is bringing about change? • Can you think of why we still lack good frameworks for implementing and evaluating clinical governance?

Audit

What is audit?

Clinical audit was defined by the Department of Health (Anon 1993: np) as involving: 'systematically looking at the procedures used for diagnosis, care and treatment, examining how associated resources are used and investigating the effect care has on the outcome and quality of life for the patient'.

Audit as an expectation preceded clinical governance. Johnston (2000) argued that as with clinical governance, the introduction of audit was based more on faith than any evidence. The concept of medical audit was first introduced in the 1989 White Paper, *Working for Patients* (DoH 1989) and funding was initially only available for doctors. In 1990 medical audit was extended to nurses and by 1993 the term 'clinical audit' was established. The initial emphasis was to examine all aspects of patient care from assessment through to outcomes. However, clinical audit has been more widely used. A less common definition is that 'audit is the process of reviewing the delivery of care to identify deficiencies so that they can be remedied'.

Clinical audit is any audit that relates to aspects of clinical service delivery. It can be carried out by a single professional or staff group or by a multi-disciplinary team (Nicol 1990). In a field such as child and adolescent mental health many of the audits are likely to involve all members of the team rather than just one professional group. Collis (2006) argues that the paucity of literature on the role of the nurse in clinical audit demonstrates that nurses are not being supported in doing audit as an integral part of their roles and that they need to demand the resources to do so.

Why audit?

The value of clinical audit (if done properly – and that is an important caveat) is that it can serve several useful functions. Perhaps the most important of these is that it provides clinical teams with the opportunity to improve the services they provide. Audit can help in the following ways:

- identifies and promotes good practice and may lead to improvements in service delivery and outcomes for service users;
- provides a focus on which areas to target to improve quality;
- ensures that service delivery and developments are truly patient-centred and genuinely involve patients;
- considers how to involve patients in planning better services;
- helps identify areas of potential risk and, enabling action to be taken to reduce such risk;
- demonstrates that services are effective and cost-efficient;
- provides opportunities for training and education;
- demonstrates the team's commitment to quality.

Example in practice

In our local CAMHS we undertook a small audit project looking at whether and how well CAMHS clinicians undertook an examination of substance misuse history in young people. We found that this was generally poorly done. We introduced a pro-forma to serve as a reminder but also used the opportunity to run two training sessions on substance misuse. When we re-audited case notes, we found that the history-taking had improved considerably.

The caveat that audit needs to be done properly is highlighted in Dogra (2003). In this study it was found that staff often considered that they were undertaking audit projects but often had no clear goals or coherent methodology.

There are also different types of audit (Nicol 1990; Hardman and Joughin 1998). Nicol uses the term 'input' while Hardman and Joughin use the term 'structure' to describe audits that look at the availability of resources and personnel. There are also process audits which focus on the various processes that take place within service delivery such as assessment, treatment or management to establish how resources within these are used. Finally there are outcome audits, which assess which changes can be attributed to the clinical intervention. In practice many of the audits that are undertaken are process audits that look at fairly superficial aspects such as whether someone got an appointment at a particular time or which forms were completed. There is relatively little focus on quality so that while audits may check if an assessment is undertaken they rarely measure whether the quality met a certain pre-agreed standard. When standards are applied they often relate to targets rather than clinical standards of delivery. Again, locally we have more audits that focus on the peripheral aspects than those that focus on the direct clinical care aspects.

In summary audit can clarify:

- whether what is said to be happening is actually happening;
- whether current performance meets existing standards;
- whether clinical practice uses the evidence available (be it from research or practice).

What does audit involve?

Hardman and Joughin (1998) offer a step-by-step guide to audit which is summarized in Table 13.1. Dogra (2003) reviewed audit activity in one UK CAMHS and this is used to provide examples.

Planning an audit

Despite availability of good guidance it can often still be difficult to carry out audit in clinical practice. Time is often cited as a reason. However, poor support and understanding can also inhibit useful audits. There may be a tendency to focus on process audits rather than those that might improve direct clinical care.

Johnston (2000) looked at the barriers and facilitators for effective clinical audit by reviewing 93 publications of audits and audit evaluation. There were five main areas under which barriers were identified:

- lack of resources;
- lack of expertise or advice in project design and analysis;

Table 13.1 The steps of an audit project

Step	Example: CAMHS service audit (Dogra 2003)
Select topic	Audit activity and standards within CAMHS
Review literature	Identified that there was little written about this
Set standards	The service should be completing audit projects that are relevant to the service and findings should be implemented
Design the audit	Survey method to identify what audit was happening and whether findings were implemented Also collected data on whether audit was useful
Collect data	Sent questionnaire to all clinicians in the services
Analyse data	Quantitative analysis – simple frequencies
Feedback findings	Many projects called 'audit' were in fact not audit There was no record of completed audits if they were completed Audit activity was rather fragmented
Change practice	Established a service-wide audit group which monitored and provided support for audit activity (including some training)
Set/review standards	The standard remained that the service should be completing audit projects that are relevant and findings should be implemented
Re-audit	Re-surveyed all clinicians with additional questions about the new forum

- problems between groups and group members;
- lack of an overall plan for audit;
- organizational impediments.

Key facilitators were:

- modern medical record systems;
- effective training;
- dedicated staff;
- protected time;
- structured programmes;
- shared dialogue between purchases and providers.

Another key finding from Johnston (2000) was that audit was not systematic or integrated into services and a significant amount of the activity was still confined to enthusiasts. It is important to recognize that for clinical staff, training is more usefully provided by someone who understands the context of their work. It is also important that the service as a whole is committed to the activity. The development of a service-wide audit group as described by Dogra (2003) sought to address many of the barriers by providing training and support. In additon, all proposed audit projects went through the audit to ensure that the methodology was sound and that the project was relevant to the service. The monitoring of the projects ensured that they were completed and findings forwarded to the clinical governance group for implementation.

Box 13.2 **Exercise**	• Reflect on how much of our discussion of audit is reflected in your organization. • How has your organization addressed any barriers?

The difference between audit and research

Clinicians may feel that audit is too much like research and so perceive it to be out of their depth. There are similarities between research and audit, so this can be a confusing area. The matter is further complicated by the fact that audits do not generally require ethics approval on the rationale that patients are usually not directly involved and that nothing 'new' is being piloted or tested. Thus research can sometimes be renamed as audit to avoid the ethics approval process.

While there are similarities and both are required to continue to develop and improve clinical services and care, there are important differences. Research will be discussed in more detail in the chapter that follows but it is worth remembering that they have different aims: research will often aim to establish new information, while this is usually not the purpose of audit.

Remarkably little appears to have been written about clinical governance and audit as they apply to CAMH. A few audit projects have been described – for example, Brown and Bruce (2004) outline an audit on the diagnosis and treatment of attention deficit hyperactivity disorder (ADHD). Several authors (Black 1992; Smith 1992; Closs and Cheater 1996) have clarified the differences between research and audit and these are summarized in Table 13.2.

There is debate about whether audit is a type of research but with a different purpose. Black (1992) describes the relationship between audit and evaluative research and highlights the fact that research itself should be subject to audit for the same reasons that clinical practice is subject to audit. Using that same logic, audit is an appropriate subject for research

Table 13.2 The differences and similarities between research and audit

	Research	**Audit**
Aims	To discover new knowledge, such as whether an intervention is effective, and cost effective	To ensure research findings are implemented; to improve clinical practice by monitoring or assessing it
Purpose	'Research is concerned with discovering the right thing to do' (Smith 1992), e.g. the effectiveness of a particular treatment	'Audit is ensuring that the right thing is done right' (Smith 1992), e.g. to measure the effectiveness of a particular service in delivering a treatment that is known to be effective
Driver	Ultimately may be to improve practice and patient experience but that is usually through increasing knowledge and understanding	Improve practice and patient experiences
Methods	Can be experimental and may test a new practice, therapy or drug	Should not be experimental: unproven treatments should not be tested for effectiveness under the guise of audit
	Can use quantitative methods such as questionnaires or qualitative methods such as semi-structured interviews or mixed methods	Can use quantitative methods such as questionnaires or qualitative methods such as semi-structured interviews or mixed methods
Sample	Sample size and selection criteria are critical	Sample size is often not important
	Can involve all types of staff and patients	Can involve all types of staff and patients
	Particular attention may need to be given to vulnerable groups, e.g. children	Vulnerable groups may need some attention
Outcomes	Generally research aims to ensure that the results are generalizable to other contexts	Generally findings are unlikely to be generalizable and this is fine. However, the methods for particular audits may be generalizable to other services especially if they are looking at the same issue
	Feedback to individual participants not usually indicated but may be part of good practice	Feedback to staff involved in audit should be integral to process to improve practice
Ethical approval	Always need to check if required or not	Usually not needed as data collection is an integral part of the care process
Consent	Always needed	Usually broad consent obtained when patient enters services
Confidentiality	Usually required if assured at outset	Patient confidentiality will need to be maintained. Individual clinician data may or may not be confidential depending on context and circumstances of audit
Training	Formal training is usually helpful	Formal training is usually helpful

(e.g. research into the methodology used in audits may help to identify better methods for future projects).

Box 13.3 Exercise	• How would you audit assessment standards within your CAMHS?

Supervision

What is supervision?

Clinical supervision is a formal process of professional support and learning which enables individual practitioners to develop knowledge and competence, assume responsibility for their own practice and enhance consumer protection and safety of care in complex situations (NHS Management Executive 1993). All nurses should be receiving regular supervision to support their practice but Fowler (1995) argues that there is not one model of supervision that will suit the needs of all nursing contexts. The choice of model will remain within individual areas that of most benefit to meet specific needs.

Supervision is a dynamic, interpersonally focused experience and promotes the development of therapeutic proficiency. One of the primary reasons for supervision is to ensure that the quality of therapeutic intervention with the client is of a consistently high standard and is appropriate for the client's needs. Consequently, supervision must be acknowledged as a cornerstone of clinical practice (Mental Health Nurses Association's Care and Practice Group 2005).

Supervision models

There are various supervision models available which can be used as a framework for nurses and can be adapted to suit different styles. Two widely used models are those of Proctor (1987) and Heron (1989).

Proctor introduced a model of supervision that originated from counselling and has three core domains which are:

- *formative* – skills and knowledge development;
- *normative* – professional accountability, maintaining and monitoring practice;
- *restorative* – stress survival, colleague/social support.

Proctor explained that both supervisor and supervisee carry some degree of responsibility for the development of students/workers (the formative task). Within the formative task the supervisee's strengths and weaknesses are assessed and assistance provided to increase knowledge and build skills and expertise. This area also enables the supervisor to monitor the supervisee's work and ensure appropriate caseloads for safe practice.

Heron's (1989) model is based on a six-category intervention analysis framework. The conceptual model was originally developed to assist in the understanding of interpersonal relationships and related to the client/practitioner. The six categories were identified as prescriptive, informative, confronting, cathartic, catalytic and supportive.

Sloan and Watson (2002) stated that *prescriptive interventions* include offering advice and making suggestions: they seek to direct the behaviour of the client. To be *informative* is to offer information or instruction. To be *confronting* is to challenge the person's behaviour, attitudes or beliefs. *Cathartic interventions* include enabling the release of tension and strong emotion – for example, grief, fear and anger. *Catalytic interventions* include encouraging further self-exploration, self-directed living, learning and problem-solving in the client. To be *supportive* is to validate or confirm the worth and value of the client's personal qualities, attitudes or actions.

It is clear that this model could be developed to work not only with practitioners and clients but also to enable the relationship between supervisor and supervisee. The interpersonal focus lends itself to the necessary essential relationship that forms the basis of effective clinical supervision.

Skills of the supervisor in CAMHS

Faugier (1998) states that supervision which is not built upon an open, trusting, positive relationship will be virtually useless. Ideally there should be some choice in relation to the identified supervisor, but practically this is not always feasible, unless the individual's therapeutic role dictates specialist knowledge related to their particular area of work. This may be particularly relevant in CAMHS where services tend to be small with more focus on the multi-disciplinary team. As in Proctor's approach the responsibility for effective supervision lies with the supervisor and supervisee. Both need to commit to the relationship and the sessions, in order that the supervision has value and purpose. The supervisor should be able to demonstrate effective interpersonal and facilitative skills. One hour a month is the minimum time that should be expected, in order to foster the development of a mutually respectful and receptive relationship between the two individuals involved to create a positive experience for both parties. It is helpful to have a regular slot in the week, which reinforces the essential requirement of supervision, rather than arranging ad hoc sessions, which are more likely to be cancelled. Supervision styles vary dependent on the individuals concerned and any particular model adopted by the service. Faugier (1998) suggests that just as one would expect the nurse to have the ability selectively to blend various clinical approaches in response to patients' needs, the supervisor should be able to demonstrate such ability during supervision. The supervision agreement should be formalized in either a written or verbal contract. While acknowledging confidentiality, some agreed means of recording the issues discussed is helpful to both supervisor and supervisee for continuity and reflection purposes.

Types of supervision

There are several types of supervision such as managerial, professional, peer and/or clinical. All types aim to benefit and enhance the promotion of personal and professional development and are often overlapping. Supervision may be offered either as a single intervention or a combined means of support. These mechanisms facilitate the development of professional practice and therapeutic proficiency, and safeguard standards of care. Supervision sessions are a confidential arena that enable nurses to reflect upon and explore their own practice in a safe environment while facilitating personal growth. Supervision should promote accountable practice and include an evaluation of the supervisee's performance, with the process being linked to the individual's personal development plan.

Box 13.4 Types of supervision

- Clinical.
- Managerial.
- Peer.

Clinical supervision

Supervision is integral and essential to competent clinical practice. It may explore particular concerns, the individual's management of their caseload and specific clinical matters. During the sessions it is useful and good practice to routinely discuss issues such as child protection, vulnerable adults and the care programme approach. This is an opportunity to raise nurses' awareness of their statutory obligations and promote safe working practice. Clinical supervision is now a fundamental component of nursing and all CAMHS nurses should expect regular, meaningful sessions as part of their contract of employment. This time will inevitably compete with the demands of their working environment and those nurses based on inpatient wards are at greater risk of supervision being cancelled due to staff shortages. While there is an acknowledgment that supervision is seen as important, patient care takes priority. This is particularly unfortunate as these areas can present difficult challenges and nurses benefit from being able to access space in which to discuss dilemmas and concerns. Being able to share and explore their emotional and practical responses to situations in a supportive environment can help nurses to manage stress more effectively. Evidence of a service's established supervision structure will be a significant influential factor in the recruitment and retention of nurses.

Managerial supervision

Managerial supervision will involve the nurse's line manager or team leader/manager. These sessions are likely to focus on managerial issues such as annual leave, on call, attendance and ill health reviews. In addition to the issues discussed in supervision, the line manager is in a position to particularly focus on professional development and explore opportunities to support the career aims of the supervisee. They should also have an understanding of their service's future developments and be in a position to consider the appropriateness and feasibility of the aspirations of the supervisee and where these might fit into the individual's personal development plan and the needs of the service. If different individuals are involved in the supervision process it is essential that the supervisors negotiate the areas to be covered to ensure that comprehensive support is in place that covers all aspects of the nurse's role.

In any one-to-one supervision the relationship between supervisor and supervisee is crucial to the therapeutic value of the sessions. There may be occasions when it is necessary to change the supervisor due to the nature of the relationship. This is not always easy to achieve in CAMHS, which tend to be small, with the likelihood of there being fewer alternative options available.

Peer supervision

Peer supervision is a useful and popular means of support and is particularly helpful when provided alongside individual supervision. Groups are self-motivated and self-managed. While the topics shared and discussed may be similar to those raised in individual sessions, the group offers a range of views and opinions and can feel very supportive to individuals, particularly as it removes the hierarchical element. In addition to being more cost effective and achievable it has been suggested that peer support has advantages over individual supervision. Butterworth and Faugier (1994) suggest that the one-to-one approach is anecdotally common, but consistently seen as problematic as it carries a high risk of encouraging collusion and provides a weak means of addressing poor practice. Severinsson (2003) talks about stress in the workplace and suggests that systematic clinical supervision or peer support, based on the principles of recovery, empowerment and self-help have proved to be an effective means of assistance.

Effectiveness of supervision

There is considerable evidence related to supervision in nursing but little that is CAMHS-specific. Most of the literature available relates to adult mental health and older persons nursing. Following an extensive evidence-based literature review, Brunero and Stein-Parbury (2007) concluded that clinical supervision provides peer support and stress relief for nurses as well as a means of promoting professional accountability, skill and knowledge. They also suggested that more research is needed into the effectiveness of clinical supervision in other specialities, one of which would be CAMHS.

Supervision is an important component of the nursing role and nurses need to understand its function as they will often be supervisors or supervisees. It is also evident that considerably more work needs to be undertaken in establishing what facilitates effective supervision in CAMHS.

Box 13.5 Exercise	The following issues could be discussed in nursing groups to enable nurses to explore and reflect upon the quality of their own supervision:

- What makes good supervision?
- Are all nurses in your organization/service accessing supervision – is it enhancing practice?
- How is the supervision structured?
- What are the skills and attributes required for a competent supervisor?
- What amount of time is allocated to supervision sessions?
- Is the supervision audited?

Summary

This chapter has focused on some key aspects of professional practice which are not direct clinical care but are closely linked to how clinical care is provided. Clinical governance, audit and supervision are not specific to CAMHS nurses and it may be because of this that nurses have yet to maximize their potential contribution in these areas. Hopefully, in reading through this chapter, you will have begun to develop ideas as to how these areas might contribute to your practice and the continued development of your professional role.

References

Anon (1993) *Clinical Audit: Meeting and Improving Standards in Healthcare*. London: Department of Health.

Balogun, J. and Hope-Hailey, V. (2004) *Exploring Strategic Change*, 2nd edn. Harlow: Prentice Hall.

Black, N. (1992) The relationship between evaluative research and audit, *Journal of Public Health Medicine*, 14(4): 361–6.

Brown, G. and Bruce, K. (2004) A nurse-led ADHD service for children and adolescents, *Nursing Times*, 100(40): 36–8.

Brunero, S. and Stein-Parbury, J. (2007) The effectiveness of clinical supervision in nursing: an evidence-based literature review, *Australian Journal of Advanced Nursing*, 25(3): 109–15.

Butterworth, T. and Faugier, J. (1994) *Clinical Supervision: A Position Paper*. Manchester: School of Nursing Studies, University of Manchester.

Closs, S.J. and Cheater, F.M. (1996) Audit or research – what is the difference? *Journal of Clinical Nursing*, 5(4): 249–56.

Collis, S. (2006) A review of the literature on the nurse role in clinical audit, *Nursing Times*, 102(12): 38.

Dogra, N. (2003) Audit of audit activity in a child and adolescent mental health service, *Clinical Child Psychology and Psychiatry*, 8(1): 27–35.

DoH (Department of Health) (1989) *Working for Patients. Working Paper 6*. London: HMSO.

Faugier, J. (1998) The supervisory relationship, in T. Butterworth, J. Faugier and P. Barnard (eds) *Clinical Supervision and Mentorship in Nursing*. Cheltenham: Nelson Thornes.

Fowler, J. (1995) Nurses' perception of the elements of good supervision, *Nursing Times*, 91(22): 33–7.

Hardman, E. and Joughin, C. (1998) *FOCUS on Clinical Audit in Child and Adolescent Mental Health Services*. London: Royal College of Psychiatrists.

Heron, J. (1989) *Six Category Intervention Analysis*. Guildford: Human Potential Resource Group, University of Surrey.

Johnston, G. (2000) Reviewing audit: barriers and facilitating factors for effective clinical audit, *Quality in Health Care*, 9: 23–36.

Mental Health Nurses Association's Care and Practice Group (2005) Clinical supervision, *Mental Health Nursing*, 13(1).

NHS Executive (1997) *Personal Medical Services: Pilots Under the NHS. A Guide to Local Evaluation*. London: DoH.

NHS Management Executive (1993) *What Does This Stand For?* Nursing and Midwifery Council A–Z Advice Sheet 2006.

Nicol, A.R. (1990) Audit in child and adolescent psychiatry, *Archives of Disease in Childhood*, 65: 353–6.

Proctor, B. (1987) *Supervision: A Cooperative Exercise in Accountability. Enabling and Ensuring Supervision in Practice*. Leicester: National Youth Bureau and the Council for Education and Training in Youth and Community Work.

RCN (Royal College of Nursing) (2003) *Clinical Governance: An RCN Resource Guide*. London: RCN.

Scally, G. and Donaldson, L. (1998) Clinical governance and the drive for quality improvement in the new NHS in England, *British Medical Journal*, 317: 61–5.

Severinsson, E. (2003) Moral stress and burnout: qualitative content analysis, *Nursing and Health Sciences*, 5: 59–66.

Sloan, G. and Watson, H. (2002) Clinical models for nursing structure, research and limitations, *Nursing Standard*, 17(4): 41–6.

Smith, R. (1992) Audit and research, *British Medical Journal*, 305: 905–6.

Thomas, M. (2002) The evidence base for clinical governance, *Journal of Evaluation in Clinical Practice*, 8(2): 251–4.

Further reading

Morrell, C. and Harvey, G. (1999) *The Clinical Audit Handbook: Improving the Quality of Health Care*. London: Balliere Tindall in association with the Royal College of Nursing.

14 Nurses and CAMH research

Sharon Leighton, Laurence Baldwin and Peter Nolan

He who does not doubt does not investigate, and he who does not investigate does not perceive, and he who does not perceive remains in blindness . . .[1]

Key features
- Identification of evidence as a driver for change and its effects on mental health nursing.
- Overview of different sources of CAMHS evidence.
- Challenges inherent in CAMH.
- The role of CAMH nurses in research.

Introduction

Despite nurses being the largest single professional group in child and adolescent mental health services (CAMHS), they are the least established with respect to academic and professional development (Welsh National Assembly 2000). If they are to attain parity with other professions within mental health care, it is imperative that they unite and agitate for much better educational opportunities than has been the case hitherto (Williams and Gale 2003). Access to relevant and appropriate training resources is now essential if health care providers are to contribute to the modernization of all health care services within the National Health Service (NHS). As CAMHS improve it is important that nurses participate in setting the parameters for research and teaching and are at the forefront of setting educational agendas and applying research in practice (Nolan 2003; Williams and Gale 2003; Leighton 2007).

This chapter provides an overview of different sources of CAMHS evidence. It aims to encourage nurses to learn more about CAMH research, its importance and how to critique the evidence. It is divided into three main sections: the need for evidence; a broad discussion on the current status of child mental health research and identified priorities (this is not confined to the UK); and the contribution of CAMH nurses to the research agenda.

The need for evidence

While the endeavour to roll out research-based practice has met with approval from some, not all have viewed this development as enthusiastically as the policy-makers. It has been claimed that the assumption that evidence can be instantly transferred into practice is naive. Wickham (1999) contends that research findings form only a part, and a relatively small part, of the toolkit of clinical decision-making and of equal, if not more importance, are careful observation

---

[1] Abu Hamid al-Ghazali (1058–1111 CE), *Confessions* or *Deliverance from Error*.

of and engagement with the patient, clinical experience and 'hunches' borne out of long experience and reflection. The fiercest critics of evidence-based practice assert that it diminishes the importance of health professionals' and patients' experiences, and can assume that findings based on samples or even on populations are directly applicable to individuals. Critics also suggest that it belittles the priorities of service users and is of no use to clinicians when the evidence is equivocal or simply not available (Smith 2003).

One might assume that services that were formalized just over a decade ago, such as CAMHS, should be in a better position to respond to 'best practice' than those with a much longer histories. Guyatt et al. (2001) assert that in order for this to happen, team members should be capable of actively participating in decision-making and committed to implanting agreed interventions. However, for services to be consistently effective, more is required than just multi-disciplinary collaboration. Collaboration between services, service users and carers is necessary so that specific issues are openly contested and consensus reached. Practitioners should ideally have current and accurate information regarding diagnoses, aetiology of illnesses, moderating factors, treatment options and side-effects, while service users have ownership of their conditions, their values, their treatment preferences and their treatment goals (Edwards and Elwyn 2001).

Evidence as a driver for change

Organizations such as The Cochrane Collaboration have laid much emphasis on frameworks, targets and guidelines as a means of transforming services. Yet by focusing predominantly on research findings, little consideration has been given to the methodological processes that underpin knowledge transfer in practice. Moreover, the research approach is open to attack in terms of reductionism, reducing health care interventions to medication, treatment techniques and information-giving, while ignoring the wider context in which service users live and which gives meaning to their lives.

The nursing perspective

From a nursing perspective, the current preoccupation with research and the evidence-based approach to care threatens mental health nurses, regardless of the type of service in which they work. Without the skills of research appraisal or enjoying confident evidence literacy, nurses, including mental health nurses, will fail to appreciate the complexity of the process of producing evidence and will be limited in their ability to participate fully in the creation of a research culture (Freshwater 2005). The optimistic vision enshrined in Project 2000 that nursing would become an all-graduate profession, based in universities, has not materialized. Currently, only 4 per cent of the nursing workforce are graduates (Shields and Watson 2007) and Holmes (2006) detects a malaise among mental health nurses related to their lack of appropriate education and the fact that much of their work is invisible and hence not measurable. Without a workforce that is research literate, the transference of good quality evidence into practice is impeded.

As a result of diminishing resources available for mental health education and training, nurses in practice settings are struggling to understand new concepts while abandoning the skills that were once considered to be fundamental to their profession (Hamilton and Roper 2006). A strong emphasis on managerialism in health care generally, and mental health care in particular, means that the role of the nurse is becoming increasingly administrative. At the end of the first decade of the twenty-first century, mental health nurses continue to find their role and status ambiguous and perhaps threatened (Handy 1991). Today, this is because a new research hierarchy among health professionals and a new managerial culture in the health service once again leave mental health services and their providers at a disadvantage.

The next section considers the research agenda in relation to CAMH.

Research into CAMH

The focus of this section is CAMH research. The aim is not to provide a summary of the evidence (although some will be included as exemplars), but to identify different types of research evidence, acknowledge priorities and some of the challenges.

Vostanis (2007) states that there have been worldwide changes in CAMHS over the past decade, with these reflected in a developing evidence base, plus practice and service innovations. Nevertheless, the majority of research studies published continues to originate from western countries and from a relatively few research organizations (WHO 2005; Patel and Kim 2007; Vostanis 2007). Overall, few countries undertake research into CAMH, few have a specific CAMH policy, and very few have a national plan for CAMH research (WHO 2005).

In the UK no national plan for research into CAMH exists at the time of writing. McCombie and Chivers (2005), who work for the National Institute for Mental Health in England (NIMHE), carried out a consultation exercise with some CAMHS professionals to identify research priorities. Priorities identified include:

- population-based approaches to mental health promotion and intervention;
- overcoming barriers to multi-agency collaborative working (e.g. in assessment, planning, intervention and training);
- access to specialist mental health services;
- developing the evidence base about extending efficacious treatments and interventions into real-world practice.

McCombie and Chivers suggest that these recommendations should not be considered as representative of all stakeholders, but be examined alongside other consultations with relevant stakeholder groups.

In January 2006 the CAMHS Evidence-Based Practice Unit (EBPU) was established. The unit aims to help professionals in developing best practice through promoting outcomes-based and evidence-informed practice (Anna Freud Centre 2008). Wolpert (2008) defines evidence-informed practice as a sequential process, involving examining evidence from the academic literature and from one's own practice and that of other clinicians. This raises a question as to how busy clinicians can access the emerging evidence base; what sources of evidence are available to peruse.

Different sources of research evidence

Leffingwell and Collins (2008) identify that CAMH clinicians often lack both the time and the resources (e.g. access to database searches or full-text copies of the literature) to make personal primary-source searches for data. They may also lack the necessary skills. However, there are an increasing number of resources available that provide credible reviews and summaries of the most current evidence. These are deemed more useful to practitioners: commissioned reviews or institute reports; clinical practice guidelines and consensus statements; Cochrane reviews; textbooks (Leffingwell and Collins 2008). Each is considered briefly.

Commissioned reviews or institute reports

Governments can commission summaries of evidence. For example, in the UK, Fonagy *et al.* (2002) were awarded a grant from the Department of Health (DoH) in order to provide a systematic review of CAMH treatment. These authors' summary of the evidence identifies large gaps in the evidence base, even in the two areas of intervention where there are relatively large numbers of randomized control trials (RCTs) – i.e. psycho-pharmological treatments and cognitive behavioural therapy (CBT) for particular childhood problems (Fonagy *et al.* 2002). The reviewers also identified several underlying assumptions and characteristics associated with research into CAMH treatment. These include: commitment to comprehensive outcomes evaluation; appreciation of the need to measure change across several domains; concern regarding the experience of users of services; concern with the generalization of outcomes across settings and time (Fonagy *et al.* 2002).

An example of an institute report is the *Truth Hurts: Report of the National Inquiry into Self-harm Among Young People* (Mental Health Foundation 2006). This was a joint inquiry, launched by the Mental Health Foundation and the Camelot Foundation, that sought to bring together all available evidence from a variety of sources in order to provide a thorough and evidence-based platform for changes in understanding, prevention of, and responses to, self-harm among young people in the UK. Recommendations include the need for robust evaluation of all types of intervention and treatments, and evaluation of any improvements to patients' experiences arising out of the National Institute for Health and Clinical Excellence (NICE) guidelines on self-harm (Mental Health Foundation 2006).

A note of caution in relation to institute reports; they are rarely peer reviewed and can be biased.

Clinical practice guidelines and consensus statements

An example of a clinical practice guideline is the NICE[2] guideline on depression in children and young people (the first mental health guideline solely for children) (NICE 2005). The research recommendations made by the Guideline Development Group, based on its review of the evidence, include: an appropriately blinded RCT to assess the efficacy and the cost-effectiveness of individual CBT, systemic family therapy and child psycho-dynamic psychotherapy compared with each other and treatment as usual; a similar RCT assessing efficacy and cost-effectiveness of fluoxetine, the favoured psychological therapy (from Phase 1), and combination of these compared to each other and placebo;[3] a qualitative study to examine the experiences in the care pathway of children and young people and their families (and perhaps professions) to inform decisions about the most appropriate pathway of care; and an appropriately designed study to compare validated screening instruments for detection of depression in children and young people (NICE 2005).

Cochrane reviews

The Cochrane Collaboration is an international not-for-profit, independent organization, devoted to providing up-to-date, accurate information about the effects of health care readily available worldwide. It produces and disseminates systematic reviews of health care interventions and promotes the search for evidence in the form of clinical trials and other studies of interventions (Cochrane Collaboration 2008).

---

[2] NICE guidelines provide recommendations for good practice based on the best available evidence of clinical and cost-effectiveness.

[3] Goodyer *et al.* (2007) report on an RCT which aimed to determine whether a combination of a selective serotonin reuptake inhibitor (SSRI) and CBT together with clinical care is more effective in the short term than an SSRI and clinical care alone in adolescents with moderate to severe major depression.

Examples of systematic reviews associated with CAMH are provided by Bower *et al.* (2001), Pratt and Woolfenden (2002), Ekeland *et al.* (2004), Merry *et al.* (2004), James *et al.* (2005), Kennedy *et al.* (2007) and Rathbone *et al.* (2008). The majority identify insufficient evidence and all highlight the need for further research.

It is worth noting that reviews undertaken by the Cochrane Collaboration assess original research, whereas commissioned reviews may review only the reviews.

Textbooks

Caution is urged when using textbooks as a sole source of evidence summaries for two main reasons: they may be biased editorially and become out of date quickly as the evidence base evolves (Leffingwell and Collins 2008).

However, such concerns do not relate solely to textbooks. For example, the Cochrane Collaboration has been accused of bias in relation to who is identified to undertake reviews and there are instances where policy has been developed on the basis of some very suspect research evidence (Glezerman 2006). Concern has also been expressed about the quality of NICE guidelines and their interpretation of the research (Hodes and Garralda 2007). Furthermore, Duncan (2008) identifies that most research about evidence-based practice is performed by the instigators of the approach being investigated.

Having identified various sources of research evidence, research in different contexts is considered.

Different contexts and categories of research

The different categories of research addressed in this section are associated with service provision and clinical research.

Service provision

Service provision reforms are politically driven rather than clinically or professionally led. Ideologically driven imperatives are based on political and economic considerations rather than research evidence, and can alter with changes in government, or even ministers. Furthermore, policy may be used to support health care that has not been fully evaluated against the evidence (Belfer 2007). However, it is important to acknowledge the challenges that are associated with wider structural changes within the global and UK health and social care systems (e.g. finite resources) (Malin 2000; Williams and Fulford 2007).

Research is identified in some recent national reviews and policies.[4] The *National Service Framework for Children* (DoH 2004) recommends in Standard 9 that:

- research is needed to determine the effectiveness of interventions used;
- innovative approaches should be encouraged and subjected to audit and evaluation;
- outcomes should be evaluated from the perspective of service users.

The DoH (2006) report on Standard 9 recommends that all services routinely audit and evaluate their work. Two studies evaluating this are reported to highlight constraints, including resource shortages, the continuing need to ensure validity of measures and the challenge of gaining satisfactory response rates from parents and young people.

---

[4] This includes the NICE guideline for depression in children and young people mentioned previously.

Meanwhile, the National CAMHS Review (DCSF 2008a) identifies that much of the research evidence is neither well understood by, nor accessible to, professionals. The review emphasizes the importance of practitioners being able to access best evidence and knowledge on outcomes.

Clinical research

Kazdin (2000) identifies that while CAMH clinical research has progressed considerably, its emphasis on technique-based questions limits significant future advances. He advocates the development of a broad plan for such research in order to establish an agenda that identifies the type of knowledge needed to develop the underpinnings of therapy. However, any plan for clinical research has limitations in that there is no one ultimate agenda; embracing any overall plan might inadvertently advocate rigid or narrowly focused research.

Eight years later, Higa and Chorpita (2008) observe that despite leading researchers in the USA having advocated moving treatment research into practice settings for over a decade, and policy-makers and funding sources encouraging rapid development of dissemination research, very little has been examined in real-world settings in the CAMH literature to date.

Meanwhile, in the UK, Wolpert (2008) identifies that there are a broad range of interventions currently being used in CAMHS for which very little is known about their effectiveness (e.g. play therapy, counselling, narrative therapy). There are also a growing number of interventions being used for which there is some evidence of efficacy from the literature, but that require more information about their validity in some UK contexts (e.g. interpersonal therapy). Wolpert suggests that the key priority is to evaluate the effectiveness of existing interventions in real-world settings.

Integrating the evidence

Williams and Fulford (2007) widen the debate further through the identification of the need for an approach to clinical decision-making that considers more than the evidence base. While evidence is central, there are other important variables involved (e.g. clinical expertise and patient values). Duncan (2008) identifies that in excess of 1,000 studies have demonstrated that the therapeutic alliance is seven times more important than the technique of the therapist. Furthermore, the largest source of change (accounting for at least 40 per cent) is accounted for by individual client variables (Duncan 2008). Therefore, evidence-based practice can be perceived as the integration of the best available research evidence with clinical expertise in the context of patient characteristics, culture, values and preferences (Williams and Fulford 2007; Duncan 2008).

Some of the current challenges associated with CAMH research are now identified.

Challenges inherent in CAMH research

These challenges are considered in terms of several parameters, as outlined below.

- *The extent of the research base:* this is still a relatively new area of research with a small database compared to adult mental health (Fonagy *et al.* 2002; Vostanis 2007; Wolpert 2008).
- *The scope of funded and published research:* the presence of different funding streams coupled with the complex interaction between the emerging evidence base and political priorities and preoccupations in a given country can prove challenging. Moreover, pressure

to implement a favoured policy before it has been evaluated can compromise attempts to establish meaningful evaluation (WHO 2005; Belfer 2007; Vostanis 2007; Wolpert 2008).

- *Generalizability:* the majority of studies in CAMH have occurred in the USA. The populations studied are not necessarily representative of the UK, and often involve specific populations with single problems (in reality there are often multiple problems). Many interventions are tested using highly supervised, monitored and trained staff. Moreover, some types of treatment have a larger evidence base (e.g. psycho-pharmacological; CBT). Furthermore, research associated with adult mental health emphasizes the importance of non-specific factors such as the therapeutic relationship, which are difficult to quantify and research (Fonagy *et al.* 2002; Duncan 2008; Higa and Chorpita 2008; Wolpert 2008).

- *Design issues:* quantitative and qualitative research methods tend to be used separately, whereas both add to the greater picture with quantitative methods used to establish associations between observable phenomena, and qualitative for making sense of individual experience (Wolpert 2008). There is a lack of agreement on which outcomes to use, leading to difficulty in comparing findings. No consensus exists on how to weigh different outcomes that might arise from different perspectives across different domains. Furthermore, there is no agreement as to what outcomes are perceived as the most important. Meanwhile, the question of how to make valid comparisons across studies where different outcomes have been used remains unresolved (Fonagy *et al.* 2002; Wolpert 2008).

- *Practice implications:* Vostanis (2007) identifies common themes from both western and developing countries. These include the establishment of child mental health and service needs, assessment and treatment offered by specialist CAMHS, maximizing the impact of primary care in different contexts, and the importance of core services and non-statutory organizations working in partnership. Training is perceived as a key issue (Vostanis 2007; Long 2008). Wolpert (2008) stresses the importance of recognizing that all research not only raises as many questions as it answers, but it is difficult to interpret and to draw conclusions from, while urging clinicians to follow their curiosity and experiment, explain and evaluate. Finally, combining the various types of practices (which are often guided by the clinician's underlying philosophical base, although this may be subconscious as opposed to a recognized way of working) brings its own challenges. Combining the different types of evidence and recognizing that values (our own and those of others) drive practice provides an opportunity to learn from the research literature and clinical practice, to take into consideration patient values and to constantly challenge our own assumptions and those of others (Williams and Fulford 2007; Wolpert 2008).

The next section focuses specifically on CAMH nurses and research.

CAMH nurses and research

There is a dearth of research both about CAMH nursing per se, and regarding research undertaken by CAMH nurses. While this is beginning to change, the lack of explicitly nurse-based research highlights the lack of an academic tradition within the speciality (Williams and Gale 2003). That there is good work being completed by CAMH nurses is evidenced anecdotally at the RCN (Royal College of Nursing) Children and Young People's Mental Health Forum bi-annual conference, with several nurses presenting excellent examples of local good practice and practice-based evidence. Yet, CAMH nurses frequently fail to disseminate these examples of good practice beyond a conference presentation, which can reach only a limited number of people. Similarly, the number of CAMH presentations at mainstream mental health nursing or other conferences is very small.[5]

This may be a reflection of both the relatively small size of the speciality and its youth (Williams and Gale 2003). While there is undoubtedly pressure on all nurses to be seen to be as productive as possible, there are also an increasing number of nursing staff for whom research is a key part of their job description and role (e.g. nurse consultants have research as a core component of their role, and, increasingly, this is a component of the clinical nurse specialist's job) (McDougall *et al.* 2006).

Obtaining ethics approval

A potential obstacle is the need to obtain ethics approval for any research project that involves NHS staff, patients or property. The National Research Ethics Service (NRES) approves such projects through a network of research ethics committees (RECs), and rightly sees public protection as one of its main functions (NRES 2008). Many nurses have had the experience of trying to submit a project through the ethics process and found it very offputting. However, the process of gaining ethics approval has recently improved, and the NRES website has a comprehensive help system to guide researchers through the process (NRES 2008). Furthermore, there is currently a plan to exclude student projects from the need for full ethics approval. Many NHS Trusts also employ research coordinators, who can prove an invaluable source of help. Difficulties aside, it is important that the scrutiny of any project be rigorous. Also, the process can be very helpful in enabling researchers to think through their methodology and methods, clarify their plans and consider the likely benefits and pitfalls.

Dissemination

Even if a CAMH nurse does complete a research project (and many do as part of coursework, if not as part of their normal duties), a further obstacle to dissemination is that there is no obvious place to publish (Baldwin 2002a). No specialist journal associated with the nursing elements of CAMH currently exists in the UK. There is the North American-based *Journal of Child and Adolescent Psychiatric Nursing*, and some British nurses have published there (e.g. McDougall 2005; Leighton 2008). The main British CAMH journals, *Child and Adolescent Mental Health* and the *Journal of Clinical Child Psychology and Psychiatry*, mainly publish contributions from psychiatrists and psychologists. Thus the option is to either publish in very specialist areas, or to seek to publish in paediatric nursing or generic mental health nursing journals such as *Paediatric Nursing* or *Mental Health Practice*. None of the above is a reason for CAMH nurses not to publish, but it does highlight the lack of ownership that many might feel towards the publication of practice-based evidence.

---

[5] For example, the 2008 Network for Psychiatric Nursing Research Conference had 47 concurrent sessions, of which only one was related to CAMHS (an evaluation of a teaching module). The 2008 RCN conference for nurses working with children and young people, described as 'aimed at individuals and agencies that provide care and support for children, young people and their families', had 40 concurrent sessions, none of which were explicitly related to children and young people's mental health.

The Importance of overcoming obstacles to research in CAMH nursing

Despite the obstacles, it is important that CAMH nurses continue to work towards developing a research culture within the speciality. An understanding of different research methods and terminology enables nurses to exercise their own critical judgement as to the validity of the advice offered. At the very least they need the skills to be able to critique other people's research, enabling them to assess its credibility, usefulness and applicability to their own practice. For example, reading a NICE guideline critically requires an understanding of the levels and the quality of the research reviewed, and an understanding of whether it is generalizable to other areas. Each NICE guideline contains details of how the research evidence is weighed and assessed (e.g. NICE 2005: 22). Additionally, the National CAMHS Support Service has published a guide to finding and understanding some of the complex research evidence (Lavis 2008).

Ways forward In CAMH nursing research

This generates a question as to what kind of research CAMH nurses can realistically engage in as a way of furthering the knowledge base, and developing a specifically nurse-based approach to CAMH. An increasing number of nurses are completing PhD-level research, and are bidding for funding for externally-funded projects. However, for the majority of nurses, the challenge is to develop practice-based research projects that create meaningful outcomes for children, young people and their families. Only by doing this will nurses be better able to articulate their own value, role and function within CAMHS (Baldwin 2002b). Many nurses are involved in audit projects (audit is covered in Chapter 13). Where audit projects identify the need to change practice, the opportunity arises to look at small-scale changes in practice. Those changes may be based on evidence from elsewhere, or they may be a development of ideas generated by nurses, other clinicians, or by the service users and carers themselves. Previously untried and novel approaches to delivering and developing new services need to be evaluated as to their effectiveness, and such evaluations in effect constitute a form of research. The essential element of what is essentially a very familiar thing, the developing of flexible services, is to bring the rigour of research methodology to such developments; being aware of what is changing, why changes are being introduced and having an effective way of measuring the how, what and why of the changes makes the difference between a research-based approach and mere trial and error. In essence, this is one form of developing practice-based evidence which should sit comfortably with nurses.

As noted above, NICE recognizes a variety of levels of research, and one of these is evidence from best practice that is agreed to be of general benefit. Increasingly, there is recognition that many practices which have not developed from the research evidence, but which have been evaluated and further developed using a research-style methodology, are of use (Roberts and McDougall 2006). Some of the issues, and their relevance for CAMH have recently been explored (DCSF 2008a, 2008b), leaning on the increasing interest in practice-based evidence for many forms of mental health practice (e.g. Margison *et al.* 2000; Lyons and McColloch 2006; Buchanan-Barker and Barker 2008). The important element is that these practices are validated using sound methods to ensure that they work in the way they are assumed to. The challenge lies in defining the difference between establishing practice-based evidence as an audit activity and developing new approaches that would constitute a research activity. While the concept of evidence-based practice is an exciting development, nurses need to be clear about the difference between audit (evaluating existing practices) and research (developing new practices) (Roberts and McDougall 2006).

Action research

Other methods that can be used include action research, which Karim (2001: 35) describes as 'a powerful means of enhancing and improving practice'. Karim's summary of the strengths and weaknesses of action research is a good one, warning, as it does, of the potentially time-consuming nature of the process (this can actually be said of most research methods). It is important to bear in mind that any project, if done thoroughly, is likely to take considerable input. An advantage of action research is the emphasis on service user participation in developing and collaborating with the process (e.g. Kilgour and Fleming 2000 highlight the input of mothers in their inquiry about parenting groups). This is important as current research strategies stress the need for service user and carer involvement in health service research. The principle of involving service users and carers in developing meaningful research questions and in designing research studies is promoted in the UK by the National Institute for Health Research (National Institute for Health Research 2008).

CAMH nurses should also consider working on joint projects with university-based staff. Many CAMH nurses have links with local academic departments, either formally, if part of their job description involves contributing to teaching and research, or informally because they have been on a course at that academic institution. Developing research partnerships this way is mutually beneficial. For CAMH staff it allows access to skills and resources that may not be available to them through their employer, and for the university it allows easier access to practice settings.

Summary

This chapter identifies that CAMHS suffers from the same problems as other mental health research in that most research is policy driven – aiming to contain costs, promote self-reliance and reduce professional dependence – while largely ignoring efficacy and cost-effectiveness. Researchers can follow funding opportunities with little regard for the building up of a body of clinical knowledge and practice which addresses need rather than shaping services. It highlights what research has been undertaken, problems associated with this, and discusses some considerations about future research. Suggestions are made as to how research could be managed better, who should be helped to undertake it, how service users and carers could be more involved, and the role of CAMH nurses in this.

Finally, readers are encouraged to complete the exercise in Box 14.1.

Box 14.1 Exercise: a critique of a qualitative and a quantitative research paper relating to child and adolescent mental health

Identify two research papers: a qualitative and a quantitative study. Use the following questions to critique each study.[6]

- How well is the research design described? Does the design appear thoughtful and appropriate? What design elements might have strengthened the study?
- Were service users or carers involved or consulted in developing the design of the study?

---

[6] References that might be of help in the process include Girden (2001) and Polit et al. (2001).

- Could the study have been strengthened by the inclusion of some quantitative/qualitative data?
- Is the setting/study group adequately described? Is the setting appropriate for the research question?
- Are sample selection procedures described? What type of sampling strategy was used?
- Was the sampling approach appropriate? Were the dimensions of the phenomenon under study accurately represented?
- Was the sample size adequate?
- How were data collected? Were multiple methods used and thoughtfully combined?
- Who collected the data? Were data collectors appropriate or was there something about them that might have undermined the collection of unbiased, high quality data?
- Where and under what circumstances were data gathered? Was the setting appropriate?
- Were other people present during data collection?
- To what risks did participants expose themselves?
- Did the collection of data place any burdens (e.g. time, stress, privacy issues) on participants? How might this have affected data quality?
- Has the researcher placed the research problem in the wider theoretical context?
- Given what we know about the topic, is this research the right next step?

References

Anna Freud Centre (2008) *Child and Adolescent Mental Health Services Evidence-Based Practice Unit (CAMHS EBPU)*, http://www.annafreudcentre.org/ebpu/, accessed 25 July 2008.

Baldwin, L. (2002a) Information sources for specialist nurses, *Paediatric Nursing*, 14(2): 20–2.

Baldwin, L. (2002b) The nursing role in out-patient child and adolescent mental health services, *Journal of Clinical Nursing*, 11: 520–5.

Belfer, M.L. (2007) Critical review of world policies for mental healthcare for children and adolescents, *Current Opinions in Psychiatry*, 20: 349–52.

Bower, P., Garralda, E., Kramer, T., Harrington, R. and Sibbald, B. (2001) The treatment of child and adolescent mental health problems in primary care: a systematic review, *Family Practice*, 18(4): 373–82, http://www.crd.york.ac.uk/crdweb/ShowRecord.asp?View=FullandID=12001002109, accessed 4 August 2008.

Buchanan-Barker, P. and Barker, P. (2008) The tidal commitments: extending the value base of mental health recovery, *Journal of Psychiatric and Mental Health Nursing*, 15: 93–100.

Cochrane Collaboration (2008) Download at http://www.cochrane.org/index.htm, accessed 4 August 2008.

DCSF (Department for Children, Schools and Families) (2008a) *Children and Young People in Mind: The Final Report of the National CAMHS Review*. London: DCSF.

DCSF (Department for Children, Schools and Families) (2008b) *An Evidence Informed Approach to Practice: How to Build your own Evidence Base. Conference Handbook: Evidence-Based Practice and Practice-Based Evidence in CAMH – Can they be Usefully Combined?* London: DoH.

DoH (Department of Health) (2004) *National Service Framework for Children, Young People and Maternity Services*. London: DoH.

DoH (Department of Health) (2006) *Promoting the Mental Health and Psychological Well-being of Children and Young People. Report on the Implementation of Standard 9 of the National Service Framework for Children, Young People and Maternity Services*. London: DoH.

Duncan, B. (2008) Evidence based practice (EBP): talking points, http://www.cypf.csip.org.uk/silo/files/ebp-pbe-conference-handbook.pdf, accessed 16 July 2008.

Edwards, A. and Elwyn, G. (2001) *Evidence-based Patient Choice*. Oxford: Oxford University Press.

Ekeland, E., Heian. F, Hagen, K.B., Abbott, J. and Nordheim, L. (2004) Exercise to improve self-esteem in children and young people, *Cochrane Database of Systematic Reviews* 2004, Issue 1, art. no. CD003683, DOI: 10.1002/14651858.CD003683.pub2, http://www.cochrane.org/reviews/en/ab003683.html, accessed 5 August 2008.

Fonagy, P., Target, M., Cottrell, D., Phillips, J. and Kurtz, Z. (2002) *What Works for Whom? A Critical Review of Treatments for Children and Adolescents*. New York: Guilford Press.

Freshwater, D. (2005) Mental health awareness: balancing the image, *Journal of Psychiatric and Mental Health Nursing*, 12: 1–2.

Girden, E.R. (2001) *Evaluating Research Articles*. London: Sage.

Glezerman, M. (2006) Five years to the term breech trial: the rise and fall of randomized controlled trials, *American Journal of Obstetrics and Gynecology*, 194: 20–5.

Goodyer, I., Dubicka, B., Wilkinson, P., Kelvin, R., Roberts, C., Byford, S., Breen, S., Ford, C., Barrett, B., Leech, A., Rothwell, J., White, L. and Harrington, R. (2007) Selective serotonin reuptake inhibitors (SSRIs) and routine specialist care with and without cognitive behaviour therapy in adolescents with major depression: randomised controlled trial, *British Medical* Journal, 335: 42–146.

Guyatt, G., Haynes, B. and Jaseschke, R. (2001) The philosophy of evidence-based medicine, in G. Guyatt and D. Rennie (eds) *User's Guide to Medical Literature: Essentials of Evidence-based Clinical Practice*. New York: American Medical Association.

Hamilton, B. and Roper, C. (2006) Troubling 'insight': power and possibilities in mental health care, *Journal of Psychiatric and Mental Health Nursing*, 13: 416–22.

Handy, J. (1991) Stress and contradiction in psychiatric nursing, *Human Relations*, 44: 39–52.

Higa, C.K. and Chorpita, B.F. (2008) Evidence-based therapies: translating research into practice, in R.G. Steele, T.D. Elkin and M.C. Roberts (eds) *Handbook of Evidence-Based Therapies for Children and Adolescents: Bridging Science and Practice*. New York: Springer.

Hodes, M. and Garralda, E. (2007) NICE guidelines on depression in children and young people: not always following the evidence, *Psychiatric Bulletin*, 31: 361–2.

Holmes, C. (2006) The slow death of psychiatric nursing: what next? *Journal of Psychiatric and Mental Health Nursing*, 13: 401–15.

James, A., Soler, A. and Weatherall, R. (2005) Cognitive behavioural therapy for anxiety disorders in children and adolescents, *Cochrane Database of Systematic Reviews* 2005, Issue 4, art. no. CD004690, DOI: 10.1002/14651858.CD004690.pub2, http://www.cochrane.org/reviews/en/ab004690.html, accessed 5 August 2008.

Karim, K. (2001) Assessing the strengths and weaknesses of action research, *Nursing Standard*, 15(26): 33–5.

Kazdin, A.E. (2000) Developing a research agenda for child and adolescent psychotherapy, *Archives of General Psychiatry*, 57: 829–34.

Kennedy, E., Kumar, A. and Datta, S.S. (2007) Antipsychotic medication for childhood-onset schizophrenia. *Cochrane Database of Systematic Reviews* 2007, Issue 3, art. no. CD004027, DOI: 10.1002/14651858.CD004027.pub2, http://www.cochrane.org/reviews/en/ab004027.html, accessed 5 August 2008.

Kilgour, C. and Fleming, V. (2000) An action research inquiry into a health visitor parenting programme for parents of pre-school children with behaviour problems, *Journal of Advanced Nursing*, 32(3): 682–8.

Lavis, P. (2008) *Knowing Where to Look: How to Find the Evidence you Need*. London: National CAMH Support Service/DoH.

Leffingwell, T.R. and Collins, J.R. (2008) Graduate training in evidence-based practice in psychology, in R.G. Steele, T.D. Elkin and M.C. Roberts (eds) *Handbook of Evidence-Based Therapies for Children and Adolescents: Bridging Science and Practice*. New York: Springer.

Leighton, S. (2007) Evolution of CAMHS and the role of specialist CAMH nurses, in J. Radcliffe and M. Dent (eds) *Dilemmas of the New Governance: Proceedings of the Dilemmas in Human Services*. International Research Conference Hosted by Staffordshire University September 2006. Stafford: Staffordshire University.

Leighton, S. (2008) Bereavement therapy with adolescents: facilitating a process of spiritual growth, *Journal of Child and Adolescent Psychiatric Nursing*, 21(7): 24–34.

Long, N. (2008) Editorial: closing the gap between research and practice: the importance of practitioner training, *Clinical Child Psychology and Psychiatry*, 13: 187–9.

Lyons, J.S. and McCulloch, J.L. (2006) Monitoring and managing outcomes in residential treatment: practice-based evidence in search of evidence-based practice, *Journal of American Academy of Child and Adolescent Psychiatry*, 45(2): 247–51.

Malin, N. (2000) Professionalism and boundaries of the formal sector, in N. Malin (ed.) *Professionalism, Boundaries and the Workplace*. London: Routledge.

Margison, F., McGrath, G., Barkham, M., Clark, J.M., Audin, K., Connell, J. and Evans, C. (2000) Measurement and psychotherapy: evidence-based practice and practice-based evidence, *British Journal of Psychiatry*, 177: 123–30.

McCombie, C. and Chivers, C. (2005) *Research in Child and Adolescent Mental Health Services: Results of Research Priority Setting Exercise*, http://www.kc.csip.org.uk, accessed 5 August 2008.

McDougall, T. (2005) Child and adolescent mental health services in the UK: nurse consultants, *Journal of Child and Adolescent Psychiatric Nursing*, 18(2): 79–83.

McDougall, T., Gale, F. and Nixon, B. (2006) Education, training and workforce development for nurses working in CAMHS, in T. McDougall (ed.) *Child and Adolescent Mental Health Nursing*. Oxford: Blackwell.

Mental Health Foundation (2006) *Truth Hurts: Report of the National Inquiry into Self-harm Among Young People*. London: Mental Health Foundation.

Merry, S., McDowell, H., Hetrick, S., Bir, J. and Muller, N. (2004) Psychological and/or educational interventions for the prevention of depression in children and adolescents, *Cochrane Database of Systematic Reviews* 2004, Issue 1, art. No. CD003380, DOI: 10.1002/14651858.CD003380.pub2, http://www.cochrane.org/reviews/en/ab003380.html, accessed 5 August 2008.

National Institute for Health Research (2008) *Good Practice in Active Public Involvement in Research*, http://www.invo.org.uk, accessed 9 September 2008.

NICE (National Institute for Health and Clinical Excellence) (2005) *Depression in Children and Young People: Identification and Management in Primary, Community and Secondary Care*. Leicester: The British Psychological Society.

Nolan, P. (2003) The history of community mental health nursing, in B. Hannigan and M. Coffey (eds) *The Handbook of Community Mental Health Nursing*. London: Routledge.

NRES (National Research Ethics Service) (2008) http://www.nres.npsa.nhs.uk/, accessed 9 September 2008.

Patel, V. and Kim, Y.R. (2007) Contribution of low- and middle-income countries to research published in leading general psychiatry journals, 2002–2004, *British Journal of Psychiatry*, 190: 77–8.

Polit, D.F., Beck, C.T. and Hungler, B.P. (2001) *Essentials of Nursing Research: Methods, Appraisal and Utilisation*, 5th edn. Philadelphia, PA: Lippincott.

Pratt, B.M. and Woolfenden, S.R. (2002) Interventions for preventing eating disorders in children and adolescents, *Cochrane Database of Systematic Reviews* 2002, Issue 2, art. no. CD002891, DOI: 10.1002/14651858.CD002891, http://www.cochrane.org/reviews/en/ab002891.html, accessed 5 August 2008.

Rathbone, J., Variend, H. and Mehta, H. (2008) Cannabis and schizophrenia, *Cochrane Database of Systematic Reviews* 2008, Issue 3, art. no. CD004837, DOI: 10.1002/14651858.CD004837.pub2, http://www.cochrane.org/reviews/en/ab004837.html, accessed 5 August 2008.

Roberts, I. and McDougall, T. (2006) Clinical covernance for specialist child and adolescent mental health nurses, in T. McDougall (ed.) *Child and Adolescent Mental Health Nursing*. Oxford: Blackwell.

Shields, L. and Watson, R. (2007) The demise of nursing in the United Kingdom: a warning for medicine, *Journal of the Royal Society of Medicine*, 100: 70–4.

Smith, W.R. (2003) An explanation of theories that guide evidence-based interventions to improve quality, *Clinical Governance*, 8: 247–54.

Vostanis, P. (2007) Child mental health services across the world: opportunities for shared learning, *Child and Adolescent Mental Health*, 12(3): 113–14.

Welsh National Assembly (2000) *Child and Adolescent Mental Health Services: Everybody's Business*. Cardiff: Welsh National Assembly.

WHO (World Health Organization) (2005) *Atlas: Child and Adolescent Mental Health Resources*. Geneva: WHO.

Wickham, S. (1999) Evidence-informed midwifery, *Midwifery Today*, 51: 42–3.

Williams, R. and Fulford, K.W.M. (2007) Evidence-based and values-based policy, management and practice in child and adolescent mental health services, *Clinical Child Psychology and Psychiatry*, 12(2): 223–42.

Williams, R. and Gale, F. (2003) Current approaches to working with children and adolescents, in B. Hannigan and M. Coffey (eds) *The Handbook of Community Mental Health Nursing*. London: Routledge.

Wolpert, M. (2008) Making evidence based practice a reality: what does it mean and can it be done? http://www.cypf.csip.org.uk/silo/files/ebp-pbe-conference-handbook.pdf, accessed 16 July 2008.

15 Developing mental health services for children and adolescents

Mervyn Townley and Richard Williams

Key features	• Historical overview.
	• Service developments in the UK in the twentieth and twenty-first centuries.
	• Contemporary challenges that affect service development.
	• Managing change.
	• Workforce development.

Introduction

This chapter presents our view of the challenges that face us all in developing mental health services for children and young people. In so doing we necessarily and deliberately touch on topics that other authors raise in this book in order to capture the wide agenda that emerges from many directions for the development by nurses of specialist child and adolescent mental health services (SCAMHS) in the UK.

We draw attention, for example, to the broad international agreement that the overarching philosophy of CAMHS should be based on working in collaborative, multi-disciplinary and multi-agency ways. The principles and approaches that we cover in this chapter apply to all professions, but we focus our discourse on the opportunities, challenges and roles for nurses in meeting these aims.

We reprise the history of the development of CAMHS in the UK in the twentieth century to assist readers to better understand the context of the many challenges that modern services face in competing against restrictions in new personnel, resources and finance. In this topic area, as so many others, history conditions the decisions we make now about future plans.

We describe some of the key issues that have already emerged in the twenty-first century and the policy framework within which service developments are taking place. Important matters that impinge on developing CAMHS concern how staff within and outside those services respond to change and how strategic leaders assist them to identify and deal with the very real challenges that are posed by change. We offer suggestions on managing those processes.

Furthermore, we are clear that the success or otherwise of service developments and their quality stand or fall on societies attending effectively to the education and training of policy-makers, strategists, planners, commissioners and service managers as well as practitioners. Therefore, we focus on educating nurses for work in CAMHS later in this chapter.

Service developments in the UK in the twentieth century

Historical overview

Histories of the early development of psychiatry and mental health services make few references to children or adolescents. The first efforts to create outpatient mental health services for children and young people in the UK are thought to stem from the development of a child guidance clinic in London in 1927. Later, more clinics were created across the UK, based on the child guidance model, in turn developed from an original American approach, so that by the end of the 1940s many local authorities provided a basic service (Black and Gowers 2005).

The evacuation of children from their homes in the cities during World War II led to services being developed that helped to meet the consequential needs of the children involved. This coincided with the birth of the National Health Service (NHS), which, by the end of the 1960s, employed most of the nation's relatively few child psychiatrists.

Development of inpatient units began during this same period. The Maudsley Hospital had an inpatient service for children from 1947. The number of inpatient units began to increase slowly from this time through to the 1960s. Ironically, the number of beds rose in the decade after 1964, and has fallen again since the mid-1970s. Concerns persist about appropriate accommodation for young people who require residential mental health services, as evidenced by the Mental Health Act 2007.

Nursing roles

The role of nurses in CAMHS started in child and adolescent inpatient care and the earliest reference to nurses working in child mental health is to the unit at the Maudsley Hospital. Barker (1974) saw nurses as the key therapeutic agents as a result of the relationships they form with the children in their care. The early adolescent units varied in their purposes, philosophies and models of care, and this had effects on the client groups that were suitable for admission to them. During the 1980s it was not uncommon for 50 per cent of an inpatient population to have, mainly, conduct problems. In the 1970s and 1980s, there were challenges about why nurses were engaged in caring for young people who were resident in the NHS away from their homes, and this was particularly the case where the units worked as modified therapeutic communities.

However, as investment in mental health inpatient care for adolescents was reduced, pro rata, in the 1980s and 1990s, the focus and purposes of inpatient units in the NHS moved towards working with young people who had disorders. Consequently, medical models of care became more dominant. Now, it is uncommon to admit young people solely on the basis of their conduct.

The roles of nurses with outpatients evolved much more slowly from the early 1970s and rather more rapidly in the last 20 years.

The developments to what are now SCAMHS resulted from two routes: development of child guidance clinics based on the roles of the local authorities' medical officers of health; and mental health services developed, mainly, from centres of academic excellence in the NHS. Debate took place throughout the 1960s, 1970s and 1980s about the roles and functions of each service and the professionals who worked within them (Hersov 1986).

In the mid-1970s, changes in the roles of the NHS and local authorities, which created new responsibilities for health authorities for the health of populations rather than the NHS being primarily concerned with managing hospitals, clinics and practices, were potentially groundbreaking. They could have moved forward what we now call SCAMHS. Instead, the changes that took place resulted in most of the medical staff at the child guidance clinics moving to the

NHS while child guidance social workers moved to the social service departments run by local authorities. This structural response to functional opportunities provided by the reform of the roles of statutory sector agencies, together with failure in many areas to grasp the new strategic planning opportunities and downturn in public finances, resulted in a failure to adequately tackle the problems in coordinating and financing CAMHS.

This dominance of structure over functional approaches to service design in the 1970s is illustrative of a repeated flaw in statutory sector planning that has persisted into the present. Nonetheless, the rapidly rising role of nurses in CAMHS over the last 20 years has been fanned by some of the perverse effects. Changes in the roles of social workers and educational psychologists, from the mid-1980s to the mid-1990s, resulted in less of their professional time being dedicated to working directly with children and to collaborative working with the professional staff of the SCAMHS. In many areas, many more posts for nurses and clinical psychologists were developed to fill the gaps and exploit opportunities. Now, nurses comprise the largest discipline in the workforce in most CAMHS (Audit Commission 1999) and many nurses now work across the full range of CAMHS settings.

Influential policies

One of the most influential publications of recent times was the report on the NHS Health Advisory Service (HAS) thematic review of CAMHS across England and Wales (NHS HAS 1995). That report has had a fundamental impact on policy across the UK and in many other countries. Those developments were consolidated and built on through policy progressions in England and Wales. In England, the *National Service Framework for Children, Young People and Maternity Services* (DoH 2004) sets an approach and standards that are intended to bring about improvements in mental health care for children, young people and their families. These are key components for delivering the, mainly English, government's policy *Every Child Matters* (DfES 2003). Significantly, new policy emerged in 2001 in Wales with the government's CAMHS strategy document *Everybody's Business* (National Assembly for Wales 2001), the first comprehensive policy for CAMHS in the UK. *Everybody's Business* covers the challenges in moving CAMHS to achieve, first, the capacity and capability of being sustainable and responsive before, second, they progress to becoming comprehensive services (Welsh Assembly Government 2003). Much subsequent Welsh governmental policy for the mental health of children and young people has built on *Everybody's Business* and the *National Service Framework for Children, Young People, and Maternity Services in Wales* (Welsh Assembly Government 2005).

The shifting landscape

There have been many developments in policy and academic and professional knowledge and skill relating to mental health care for minors, but also a number of influential structural NHS changes in recent years that have impacted on the delivery of SCAMHS and the roles of nurses and all other professionals within them.

Together We Stand (NHS HAS 1995) promoted better understanding of the gaps in titrating need against service provision. That report proposed a four-tier approach to aligning responses provided for children and young people to the level, frequency, complication and complexity of their mental health needs. It emphasized the importance of the links between the tiers of service and took a strategic and functional rather than a structural approach. This approach has been successful beyond the expectations of the report's authors and it is now firmly embedded in the philosophy of policy and service delivery across Wales and England as the review of CAMHS in England opines (DCSF/DoH 2008a, 2008b). It has become particularly important in promoting development of a more comprehensive range of services for children and young people in the last 14 years.

New services

New services include, for example, development of: a large number of primary mental health workers (another core HAS proposal) (Gale and Vostanis 2003, 2005; Brazier and Gale 2005); substance misuse services (NHS HAS 2006); forensic mental health services (Williams 2004; Bailey and Williams 2005); and learning disability services. However, it is arguable that, in some parts of the UK, implementation of *Together We Stand* has focused on structural rather than strategic and functional interpretations of the recommendations of the NHS HAS. In some places, this has led to confusion about the advantages of separating the functions (though not necessarily the structures) that lie within Tiers 2 and 3. This finding stresses the importance of practitioners and opinion-leaders as well as service and professional leaders and managers receiving good strategic managerial training that sits well alongside their continuing professional education. They must differentiate the functions that are required of services from the structures that are best employed to deliver them locally if service design is to reflect population needs.

Presently, there are major concerns are about the age range of SCAMHS, the transition of young people from services that are intended for adolescents to mental health services for adults, the use of inpatient beds that are intended for adults, and links with paediatric services, particularly paediatric admission wards. Each of these matters poses a number of changes and challenges for nurses who work in SCAMHS.

Nursing roles

The history outlined at the outset has influenced the relationships within and the structures of teams and the roles of nurses. Until recently, nurses with a Registered Mental Nurse qualification were the majority of recruits to nursing in CAMHS and it was not until the mid-1990s that this began to change. Now, services recognize the importance of a wider range of skills and nurses who have other qualifications (in particular in children's nursing and learning disability nursing) are contributing fully within CAMHS.

Current services emphasize the skills that staff bring and how they can contribute to the overall skill mix rather than their initial registration. This approach makes good sense given the minimal level of input in all pre-registration programmes (Hooton 1999) about the skills that are required to work with children and young people, and the service context of the expanding therapeutic needs of children, young people and families.

A significant shift away from the medical model has occurred in many CAMHS and nursing has become a more autonomous profession. New ways of working in mental health are well exemplified by many SCAMHS (Williams 2005).

Increasingly over the last 15 years nurses have been taking leading roles in providing a very wide range of service functions which we think are of particular importance for providing more equitable access to SCAMHS. They include nurses becoming: community psychiatric nurses; primary mental health workers; therapists; specialist practitioners outposted to youth offending teams; and core members of services for young people who misuse substances.

In addition, many nurses provide liaison activities and advisory functions and are involved in developing protocols for these functions. There are also nurse-led services for young people who harm themselves (Armstrong 2006), children, young people who have attention deficit hyperactivity disorder (ADHD) (Ryan 2006) and some inpatient units. Recently, various evidence-based sources, including the National Institute for Health and Clinical Excellence

(NICE), for example, have advocated use of cognitive behavioural therapy (CBT) with children and young people (e.g. NICE 2004, 2005) as a first-line specialist approach. Nurses have responded by developing skills to deliver these and other therapies including family therapy, parent training and dialectical behaviour therapy (DBT).

Specialist nursing roles

A number of roles for clinical specialists have emerged in a variety of clinical settings within CAMHS in the UK, and with a range of client groups. Consequently, there is a growing body of expertise in some areas of clinical practice. Formation of the UK ADHD Nurses Network (UKANN) has, for example, brought together a large number of clinical specialists, as well as other interested parties. Nonetheless, the nature and roles of nurses who are employed as clinical specialists is currently the subject of professional debate. There is strong opinion that nurses should have academic as well as clinical skills within the speciality if they are to have these jobs (Sparacino 2005).

Developing services in the UK in the twenty-first century

Developing policy

CAMHS only work effectively if there has been anticipation of the population's needs, understanding of the dynamic shifts that occur with the passage of time, and clarity about how the roles of generic and specialist CAMHS relate to other services that offer assistance for children and young people.

Achieving developments towards well-integrated mental health services for children and young people requires that lessons learned through research and experience are translated in integrated ways into policy at four levels. These levels are:

1 governance policies;
2 strategic policies for service design;
3 service delivery policies; and
4 policies for good clinical practice.

Governance policies, relating to how countries, regions and counties are governed, are required that set the purposes, aims and objectives for CAMHS. They should specify the need for integrated, cross-sectoral services to be designed, developed and delivered.

Strategic policies are required that translate imperatives contained in governance policies into the intent and direction of plans overall and the development of specific service components. The responsible authorities should bring together evidence from research with their knowledge and experience of the populations they serve and their profile of risks, to design services through which to discharge the political imperatives and then mount programmes for managing the performance of those services to meet the objectives that are identified for them.

Service delivery policies concern how particular services function and relate to their partner services and how affected populations are guided into and through them according to the evidence and awareness of the preferences of people who are likely to use them. Therefore, service delivery policies include evidence- and values-based models of care (Williams and Fulford 2007), care pathways and protocols and guidelines for care as well as processes for demand management, audit, review and clinical governance (Williams *et al.* 2005).

Policies for good clinical practice concern how clinical staff take account of the needs and preferences of particular patients, how they deploy their clinical skills, and the use of their work with patients to decide how guidelines, care pathways and protocols are to be interpreted in particular cases.

Each of these four aspects of policy should be influenced by the various forms of evidence that are available from a range of sources. Furthermore, policy at each level should be ethical. There are important roles for practitioners who are skilled in the mental health care of children and young people to provide advice to the authorities as they develop each of these aspects of policy.

Contemporary challenges that affect service development

Our historical summary shows how the numbers of nurses working in CAMHS have risen rapidly and their roles broadened over a short period. Now, it is apparent that nurses have very important contributions to make in designing and managing as well as delivering mental health care; they can and should have roles in developing policy and shaping CAMHS. In particular, nurses are well placed to influence service delivery policies and policies for good clinical practice. However, before they do so, their training and experience should be expanded to include aspects of operational and strategic management.

There are a number of challenges, which Shooter and Lagier (2005) refer to as the 10 pressures for change, and they provide important considerations for setting policy and management agendas for developing CAMHS. These and other pressures create opportunities for service development, but also challenges in formulating the most appropriate strategic plans. They are, therefore, important to nurses and the direction of their development as a profession and personally.

The pressures for change

1   The increasing demand on services that increases year-on-year and may not necessarily be in numerical terms, but include changes in the balance of the complexity and severity of people's problems. A big challenge is prioritizing who receives a service with the limited resources available (Williams *et al.* 2005). Shooter and Lagier (2005) make the important point that the responsibility for responding to pressures to reduce waiting times should be firmly placed on commissioners, planners and funders, and not on clinicians.

2   The ways in which changes occur within and are (or are not) negotiated between allied services also exerts pressure. The demands on social service departments, for example, are great, given their rising statutory responsibilities. Consequently, their roles in working with minors who have mental health problems and disorders have diminished in the last 30 years and this has had knock-on effects on and affected the expectations that fall on other services. It is too often the case that these changes are not overtly negotiated at strategic or operational levels.

3   Pressure also comes from political imperatives. Since the 1990s, CAMH has been on politicians' agendas in England and Wales. This is reflected in policy developments, the National Service Frameworks in both England and Wales, and public sector targets. These matters acknowledge the importance of mental health for the UK's next generation even if monies made available do not allow all interventions that could be offered to be delivered through existing services.

4   There is also pressure for change that comes from changes in the roles and values of practitioners. As nurses have become more skilled in a range of therapies and management roles, there have been consequences for their relationships with other professionals whose roles have shifted too.

5   Other pressures arise from empowering service users and their carers. While there is still a long way to go before children, young people and families have a proper say in how services

are run, their views are becoming more influential in service development. The pressure from the increasing number of incidents, complaints and investigations arguably indicates that services have a way to go before they reach users' expectations.

6 Next is the pressure that arises from external reviews that can come from professional colleges, government departments or in the form of external audit services (e.g. The Quality Improvement Network for Multi-Agency CAMHS, QINMAC, and the Quality Network for Inpatient Child and Adolescent Mental Health Services, QNIC) or regulatory services (the National Audit Office, Welsh Audit Office, Healthcare Commission and Healthcare Inspectorate Wales). They have positive influences on services, but also create pressure on performance.

7 Perhaps the most recurring theme is the pressure that derives from recurrent recon-figurations of service structures. As regards SCAMHS, we also identify changes in the organ-izations that host the NHS components. Mental health services for adults, child health services, community services and maternity services have all hosted NHS-funded SCAMHS: the configuration depends on where you live and this is particularly the case in England where some SCAMHS are managed by mental health Trusts and others are managed by acute Trusts or foundation Trusts.

8 All health care appears to be under continuous change in the way in which services are structured and some services such as SCAMHS seem to be moved, or lurch from one direct-orate, division, Trust etc. to another at intervals. All too often, the rationale for these moves is not clear to the practitioners and they make consistency of planning and service devel-opments difficult. Often, it is these recurrent changes, sometimes after short intervals, that create pressure rather than the particular part of the NHS within which SCAMHS are man-aged. Mental health services require long-term relationships between key persons in com-missioning, planning and delivery if they are to deal effectively with the real needs of populations. There is also the issue of how policies are consulted on and information pro-vided in both directions across the four levels of policy.

9 Growth of a culture of blame when things go wrong is a particular pressure. While most public bodies say that they wish to see a blame-free approach to raising the quality of services and that they recognize that not all risks can be managed, this is far from being borne out in practice. The result is pressure on clinicians to manage risk better and defen-sive approaches to referral during times of uncertainty.

10 The last pressure identified by Shooter and Lagier concerns patterns of commissioning. Arguably, commissioning of CAMHS has been slow to develop and there is still too little knowledge of CAMHS in commissioning and funding agencies. Additionally, rushed bid-ding for, sometimes non-recurrent, monies and commissioning processes that appear unsatisfactorily disjointed create pressure. This is one reason why the internal market in state-funded health care has been dismantled in Scotland and Wales.

We assert that a matter of particular importance to developing policy, services and delivering better mental health care is for the persons involved to agree from the outset of their relation-ship about the nature of the problems with which they are concerned and the roles of each agency and team within the spectrum of care that is required to deal effectively with the needs of their population.

Managing change

During the past 20 years, SCAMHS have 'grown like Topsy' (Shooter and Lagier 2005). Many services have relied on opportunities that arise with little planning and forethought to increase staff from various professions and, often, funding has been from a range of sources from within and outside the NHS. Shooter and Lagier have identified a number of matters as among the hallmarks of poor strategic and operational practice. They contribute to the pressures identified and are also reflected in tensions between strategic and operational policies and good standards of clinical practice. They are:

- vague service aims;
- lack of management;
- confused roles and responsibilities;
- weak internal communication;
- poor record-keeping;
- idiosyncratic clinical practice;
- indecisive service remit;
- unclear referral pathways;
- audit aversion;
- precarious commissioning.

Many services do not have clear service aims that give clear messages on what should be their distinctive contribution to effective CAMHS overall. SCAMHS is often the commissioning and operational management responsibility of people who have little knowledge and understanding of mental health care and this can lead to poor management practice.

Staff teams in SCAMHS usually consist of people from a range of professions. Team members may have overlapping skills, such as the ability to use a particular therapeutic approach (e.g. CBT) or assess young people who have harmed themselves. Sometimes, this can create confusion about the roles that particular people have within the teams. Also, there are significant differences in the salaries of the professional groups, which may be engaged in similar work. It is not uncommon to find skilled practitioners engaged in various administration tasks that could be performed as well by other people to the detriment of the effective use of the unique skills of these practitioners. Therefore, it is important to consider how resources are allocated to ensure the most appropriate distribution of services.

The success of good team working turns on good communication and there have been a number of reports over recent times (e.g. DCSF/DoH 2008a, 2008b) that highlight the distance we still have to go in this respect. Services that are comprised of several small teams and various professions have to work hard to ensure that good communication pathways exist. Linked closely to this is the importance of good record-keeping and audits of notes indicate this is not a particular strength of many practitioners.

Unless service solutions to problems of demand and specialization are related to the needs of the patients, there is a risk that local preferences for service structures may contribute to, rather than resolve, the availability of inequitable service functions. Similarly, the range of therapeutic approaches available to all children, young people and families may vary according to the backgrounds of particular practitioners. This may result in differences between teams in the same service. However, as the evidence for various practices increases, these variations should decrease.

An appropriate range of local and other factors could and should influence operational practice, but referrers need clear guidance about when to call on SCAMHS appropriately. Similarly, there should be agreed pathways for referral and agreed processes. We identify the importance of addressing the equity, quality and comprehensiveness of CAMH care through developments at strategic and operational policy levels.

As highlighted in Chapter 13, there is a great deal more audit activity taking place now than a decade ago, though there is still a reluctance to engage in it.

Nurses are especially well placed to advise on minimizing the challenges and disruptions that are presented by the matters we raise here. Senior nurses have key roles in developing relationships with other senior nurses within whichever part of the health system they find themselves. This is important for ensuring proper reporting and support mechanisms are in place as well as for ensuring that senior nurses within health care organizations understand the needs and demands on generic and SCAMHS.

Developing the workforce

Workforce design

Earlier, we stressed the importance of plans to develop the workforce to success in developing services and this is especially the case for SCAMHS because they are much more dependant for their quality, responsiveness and comprehensiveness on the skills of the staff rather than highly technological and expensive facilities. Nixon (2005) has reviewed workforce matters concerning CAMHS and identified a number of challenges that should be addressed. If we do so, solutions to the problems that we have outlined may open up.

The first issue is to improve workforce design and planning through a combination of local, regional and national planning. Developing an effective workforce requires clarity about putting the needs of children, young people and families at the centre of concern by identifying the skills that should meet those needs and people's preferences. Workforce plans must involve all relevant agencies. It is important to consider the skill mixes that are required and any professional conflicts should be apprehended and resolved. Sometimes, staff find change from traditional roles and functions difficult, but failure to recognize mismatches between service requirements and professional functions hinders progress in developing services effectively. Nurses who work in SCAMHS have found changes in their professional identities particularly challenging, though they have often led the way in a number of services. One of the difficulties in the past has been a lack of supporting information, but this is changing with mapping exercises.

Recruiting and retaining staff

A second topic concerns the requirement for innovation in recruiting and retaining staff. Often, SCAMHS provide good examples of innovative service developments that include introducing primary mental health workers and the other roles listed earlier. Nonetheless, recruitment of staff to these posts has been from an existing pool of staff in some services and this has had the unintended effect overall of redistributing rather than expanding the staff and expertise. The cost is depletion of other service components of experienced staff. We agree with Nixon (2005) that recruitment practices should be innovative. There are problems in training enough professionals, including mental health nurses, to meet projections of future demand. Furthermore, the present workforce is ageing. In addition, attention to retaining staff is important. To this end, robust frameworks for career progression are necessary and this is particularly important for nurses who form the largest part of the SCAMHS workforce.

It is important to make progress with new ways of working across existing professional boundaries. This approach has been policy in Wales for around four years. However, most coordinated progress has been made in England where there are number of specific projects in progress presently. They are exploring changes in services and in roles of staff in order that the needs of children, young people and families are better met. This conceptual approach also emphasizes the support and flexibility that staff require if they are to embrace change.

Another challenge is to be able to create new roles by recruiting staff from populations that have not been utilized in the past. But it is important to do this in ways that complement and do not conflict with the preferences of existing staff.

Leadership and management

Developing leadership and management skills at appropriate levels within the SCAMHS workforce is vital. Good leadership is required, for example, to overcome historical ways of working that may, sometimes, be barriers to developing new ways of working, while ensuring that what is effective is retained. Too often, leaders emerge in services by default of tasks being attached to particular posts rather than as a cohesive strategy whereby clear responsibilities are identified with the aim of translating policy and strategy into practice through appointing people who have the requisite abilities and volition. Delivery of SCAMHS requires numerous professions and agencies to be involved in coordinated care programming and practice. Good leadership is required to ensure that the hurdles are tackled and to enable particular people to work to their potential and gain satisfaction from doing difficult jobs well. Good management is required to ensure services respond appropriately, equitably, ethically and efficiently to the challenges with which they are presented and that the necessary resources, including training, are made available.

The education and training agenda

Nixon's fifth challenge for developing the existing workforce concerns changes in its pre- and post-registration education. In order to play a full role in achieving modern services, nurses must develop contemporarily appropriate expertise and skills at pre- and post-registration levels. Current preparation of nurses for work in SCAMHS is acknowledged widely to be poor and, often, the educational initiatives that do exist are not consistent across educational providers. The kernel of our advice is that educationalists should create meaningful courses that meet the real needs of all staff including, particularly, nurses, if the core competencies required are to be matched with the requirements posed by service development plans in ways that are consistent across the UK.

The challenge is to train nurses to develop expertise and skills at pre- and post-registration levels. This is because, presently, few of them acquire skills in children's mental health care before they qualify. While all specialisms could argue the same point, we believe that the challenges relating to the mental health of children are different. The reason for this is embedded in the philosophy of CAMHS being 'everybody's business'; children and young people in all settings have mental health needs. Furthermore, we argue strongly that nurses who work in every specialism are likely to be greatly assisted in their work by gaining better awareness of human psycho-social and biological development. Some higher educational establishments are attempting to address this problem, but most offer little within their curricula.

Developing core skills

In England, Skills for Health has been working to define the core functions of SCAMHS and match them against national occupational standards (Skills for Health/CSIP and NIMHE 2008). In Scotland, NHS Education for Scotland has taken a different approach by producing a 'New-to-CAMHS Teaching Package' (Heads up Scotland nd). While neither a set of standards nor competencies, this package provides a clear idea of the knowledge and skills that staff require when they work in SCAMHS. We advise use of a combination of these approaches.

Another of the challenges in providing realistic training for nurses lies in the broad range of specialisms in which SCAMHS and, therefore, nurses are engaged. There is also the tension between the desire to increase skills and knowledge within the specialism and the need to ensure educational pathways are achieved. This has become particularly evident with the introduction of Agenda for Change, which attaches importance to the levels at which staff have achieved academically when bandings are decided.

There is an established principle that all nurses should receive clinical supervision and this is firmly supported by the Nursing and Midwifery Council (NMC 2006: 1). Nurses who work in SCAMHS are no exception to this. They should have time protected by clear statements in their job descriptions if they are to receive the supervision that is necessary.

In our opinion, there are additional skills that nurses should learn as services develop. Now, a significant part of the work of all staff in SCAMHS is liaison and consultation with other professionals who work in the statutory and third sector agencies (see Brazier and Gale 2005). Training and educational programmes should ensure that the skills for liaison and consultation are included in the training that is made available.

Where are we now?

Despite the clarity of our own and others' recommendations, we are concerned about the training that is offered by SCAMHS to nurses. At present, our experience is that the education and training of nurses in SCAMHS is often chaotic and there is little evidence of coordinated training plans (RCN 2004; Baldwin 2005).

Perhaps the single most important reason behind the lack of proper training strategies is that, historically, many services have had no budget or a tiny budget that is allocated to training nurses and this is by no means isolated to SCAMHS.

These and other concerns were identified by the Care Services Improvement Partnership (CSIP) in England within the following principles of training:

All education and training should facilitate the development of a unified culture for CAMHS with true inter-agency working, the education and professional development provided for staff must be accessible and useful, at all levels from unqualified support staff to professionally qualified workers. The structure within which professional development will be provided will therefore need to be flexible. It will need to be based upon a common core framework of knowledge, skills and attitudes and that can be delivered as a module or modules.

(CSIP undated)

Research by Edwards et al. (2008) found further evidence of the difficulties that occur with training the staff of SCAMHS. They interviewed stakeholders in SCAMHS with the aim of establishing the key factors that facilitate and limit training. Their work identified seven themes that are important in bridging the gaps in knowledge, skills and attitudes of staff in CAMHS. These factors provide a useful framework for considering education and training needs.

Key themes

1 The first is strong leadership and this has been mentioned earlier in a different context. The research suggests that, rather than simply playing a gatekeeping role to training opportunities, managers should have a role in supporting staff to undertake and implement training.

2 This links closely with the importance of having a training strategy within services. Edwards *et al.* advise that there should be a stronger focus on service needs rather than needs of particular members of staff when deciding on training strategies.

3 The third theme identified was the lack of experience and training of staff, particularly prior to their entering posts in SCAMHS. Predictably, lack of resources was another theme. It is not uncommon for there to be no budget or a very small budget for inservice training purposes. In times of hardship, it is our experience that, too often, the training monies are cut first. This also creates problems when some professional groups are not restrained in the same way as others and there is disparity of training opportunities.

4 Planners and commissioners must invest in training to ensure the sustained and rising quality of the providers' work. It is also vital for staff retention.

5 The link between training and the subsequent impact on children, young people and families was another theme that Edwards *et al.* identified. Some stakeholders offered the opinion that some staff undertake various training experiences, but with no clear outcomes as regards changes to their practice. Clearly, this does not represent wise use of precious resources. A related experience presented to the researchers was that, sometimes, training gives practitioners the tools for change, but that this is resisted by colleagues. Clearer strategic understanding of the purpose of the training should help with this.

6 Finally, the research identified a number of problems regarding availability and accessibility of training. Some universities offer modules of various lengths and at different academic levels; some are skills based, while others are purely theoretical.

We conclude that more consistent approaches to training for staff who work in CAMHS in the UK are required and not solely for nurses but for all professional staff, and that future development of CAMHS is related to creating and delivering the training agenda.

Summary

Over the last century, there have been considerable changes in the services that endeavour to meet the mental health needs of children, young people and families. This chapter has focused particularly on the changing roles of SCAMHS in the UK. Looking back, we can see to what an amazing degree services have changed despite a sensation of challenge and of slow movement forward that we all experience. But there is no room for complacency; inequities and inequalities remain.

It is important that services are responsive to the needs of the populations they serve and the evidence is clear that these needs are not static. We have portrayed particularly rapid changes in the roles of nurses in this field and see that profession as having a bright and leading role in developing CAMHS in the future. There are very important tasks in which nurses should become more involved at all four levels of policy development and its implementation. Many nurses have contributions to make at Levels 3 (service delivery policies) and 4 (policies for good clinical practice). More senior nurses should also aspire to roles and increasing influence at Level 2 (strategic policies for service design) and at Level 1 (influencing government policy).

We see education and training as the keys to service development and dealing with the challenges posed by Shooter and Lagier (2005) and Nixon (2005). We have identified an agenda for training and set against it the findings of the research by Edwards *et al.* (2008).

There is a very clear value that runs throughout this chapter: the continuing ambition of providing services that meet the needs and preferences of children and young people and their families. We must find out what these needs are through proper governance channels and ensure that services keep up with them if we are to develop CAMHS appropriately and well.

References

Armstrong, M. (2006) Self-harm, young people and nursing, in T. McDougall (ed.) *Child and Adolescent Health Nursing*. Oxford: Blackwell.

Audit Commission (1999) *Children in Mind: Child and Adolescent Mental Health Services*. London: Audit Commission.

Bailey, S. and Williams, R. (2005) Forensic mental health services for children and adolescents, in R. Williams and M. Kerfoot (eds) *Child and Adolescent Mental Health Services: Strategy, Planning, Delivery and Evaluation*. Oxford: Oxford University Press.

Baldwin, L. (2005) Multidisciplinary post-registered education in child and adolescent mental health services. *Nurse Education Today*, 25(1): 17–22.

Barker, P. (ed.) (1974) *The Residential Psychiatric Treatment of Children*. London: Crosby, Lockwood & Staples.

Black, D. and Gowers, S.G. (2005) A brief history of child and adolescent psychiatry, in S.G. Gowers (ed.) *Seminars in Child and Adolescent Psychiatry*. London: Royal College of Psychiatrists.

Brazier, A. and Gale, F. (2005) Consultation: more than talking about talking? in R. Williams and M. Kerfoot (eds) *Child and Adolescent Mental Health Services: Strategy, Planning, Delivery and Evaluation*. Oxford: Oxford University Press.

CSIP (Care Services Improvement Partnership) (nd) www.cypf.csip.org.uk/camhs/workforce/education-and-training.html, accessed 7 October 2008.

DCSF/DoH (Department for Children, Schools and Families/Department of Health) (2008a) *National CAMHS Review: Interim Report*. London: DCSF.

DCSF/DoH (Department for Children, Schools and Families/Department of Health) (2008b) *Children and Young People in Mind: The Final Report of the National CAMHS Review*. London: DCSF.

DfES (Department for Education and Skills) (2003) *Every Child Matters*. London: The Stationery Office.

DoH (Department of Health) (2004) *National Service Framework for Children, Young People and Maternity Services*. London: DoH.

Edwards, R., Williams, R., Dogra, N., O'Reilly, M. and Vostanis, P. (2008) Facilitating and limiting factors of training available to staff of specialist CAMHS, *The Journal of Mental Health Training, Education and Practice*, 3(3): 22–31.

Gale, F. and Vostanis, P. (2003) The primary mental health worker within child and adolescent mental health services, *Clinical Child Psychology and Psychiatry*, 8(2): 227–40.

Gale, F. and Vostanis, P. (2005) Case study: the primary mental health team – Leicester, Leicestershire and Rutland CAMHS, in R. Williams and M. Kerfoot (eds) *Child and Adolescent Mental Health Services: Strategy, Planning, Delivery and Evaluation*. Oxford: Oxford University Press.

Hersov, L. (1986) Child psychiatry in Britain: the last 30 years, *Journal of Child Psychology and Psychiatry*, 27: 781–801.

Heads up Scotland (nd) *National Project for Children and Young People's Mental Health*, New-to-CAMHS Teaching Package, www.headsupscotland.co.uk/whatnew.html, accessed 3 July 2009.

Hooton, S. (1999) *Results of a Survey to Establish the Degree to which Pre-Registration Programmes Address Child and Adolescent Mental Health*. London: ENB.

National Assembly for Wales (2001) *Everybody's Business: Child and Adolescent Mental Health Services in Wales: Strategy Document*. Cardiff: National Assembly for Wales.

NHS HAS (Health Advisory Service) (1995) *Review of Child and Adolescent Mental Health Services: Together We Stand*. London: The Stationery Office.

NHS HAS (Health Advisory Service) (2006) *The Substance of Young Needs*. London: The Stationery Office.

NICE (National Institute for Health and Clinical Excellence) (2004) *Eating Disorders*. London: British Psychological Society.

NICE (National Institute for Health and Clinical Excellence) (2005) *Depression in Children and Young People*. London: British Psychological Society and The Royal College of Psychiatrists.

Nixon, B. (2005) *Delivering Workforce Capacity, Capability and Sustainability in Child and Adolescent Mental Health Services*. Manchester: Greater Manchester Strategic Health Authority Northwest.

NMC (Nursing and Midwifery Council) (2006) *A–Z Advice Sheet C, Clinical Supervision*. London: NMC.

RCN (Royal College of Nursing) (2004) *The Post-Registration Education and Training Needs of Nurses Working with Children and Young People with Mental Health Problems in the UK*. London: RCN.

Ryan, N. (2006) Nursing children and young people with attention deficit hyperactivity disorder, in T. McDougall (ed.) *Child and Adolescent Health Nursing*. Oxford: Blackwell.

Shooter, M. and Lagier, A. (2005) Child and adolescent mental health services – roles, functions, and management in an era of change, in R. Williams and M. Kerfoot (eds) *Child and Adolescent Mental Health Services: Strategy, Planning, Delivery and Evaluation*. Oxford: Oxford University Press.

Skills for Health, CSPI (Care Services Improvement Partnership) and NIMHE (National Institute for Mental Health in England) (2008) *National Occupational Standards. Core Functions Child and Adolescent Mental Health Services Tiers 3 and 4*. Accessed on 21 August 2009 at http://skillsforhealth.org.uk/~/media/Resource-Library/PDF/CAMHS-corefunctions.ashx.

Sparacino, P.S.A. (2005) The clinical nurse specialist, in A.B. Hamric, J.A. Spross and C.M. Hanson (eds) *Advanced Practice Nursing; An Integrative Approach*, 3rd edn. St Louis, MO: Elsevier Saunders.

Welsh Assembly Government (2003) WHC (2003) *063: NHS Planning and Commissioning Guidance*. Cardiff: Welsh Assembly Government.

Welsh Assembly Government (2005) *National Service Framework for Children, Young People, and Maternity Services in Wales*. Cardiff: Welsh Assembly Government.

Williams, R. (2004) A strategic approach to commissioning and delivering forensic child and adolescent mental health services, in S. Bailey and M. Dolan (eds) *Adolescent Forensic Psychiatry*. London: Butterworth-Heinemann.

Williams, R. (2005) Professional capability: evidence- and values-based frameworks for psychiatrists and mental health services, *Current Opinion in Psychiatry*, 18: 361–9.

Williams, R. and Fulford, K.W.M. (2007) Values-based and evidence-based policy, management and practice in child and adolescent mental health services, *Clinical Child Psychology and Psychiatry*, 12: 223–42.

Williams, R., Rawlinson, S., Davies, O. and Barber, W. (2005) Demand for and use of public sector child and adolescent mental health services, in R. Williams and M. Kerfoot (eds) *Child and Adolescent Mental Health Services: Strategy, Planning, Delivery and Evaluation*. Oxford: Oxford University Press.

Further reading

Williams, R. and Kerfoot, M. (eds) *Child and Adolescent Mental Health Services: Strategy, Planning, Delivery and Evaluation*. Oxford: Oxford University Press.

Index

INTRODUCTION TO MENTAL HEALTH NURSING

Nick Wrycraft

Full of insights into what it's like to be a mental health nursing student, including direct quotes from current students!

This engaging new textbook provides a student focused introduction to the main issues and themes in mental health nursing. The book requires no previous knowledge and the content has been carefully chosen to reflect the most significant aspects of this important and rewarding area of nursing.

The book includes specific chapters on:

- Social inclusion and the Ten Essential Shared Capabilities.
- Mental health promotion
- Mental health at different stages of the life course
- Physical health issues in mental health settings
- Mental health law
- Therapeutic interventions, specifically Cognitive Behavioural Therapy (CBT) and psychoanalytic/psychodynamic approaches
- The concept of recovery

Scenarios and exercises are used to demonstrate integration of theory and practice. These can be easily linked to your placement experience and overall learning and development. Readers are encouraged to develop an analytical and investigative approach to their studies.

Other important areas covered in the book include the National Service Framework (NSF) for Mental Health, the Care Programme Approach (CPA) and the Tidal Model of mental health nursing.

Introduction to Mental Health Nursing is the perfect introduction for all nursing students with an interest in a career in mental health nursing.

Contributors: *Geoffrey Amoateng, Amanda Blackhall, Alyson Buck, David A. Hingley, David Dean Holyoake, Richard Khoo, Mark McGrath, Mary Northrop, Tim Schafer, Julie Teatheredge, James Trueman, Henck Van- Bilsen, Steve Wood.*

Contents:
Background to mental health nurse training - Learning on practice placements - Mental health and recognition of mental illness - Risk assessment: Practicing accountably and responsibly - Mental Health Nursing and the Law - Mental health promotion - Section 2 - Children and adolescent mental health - Adult mental health services in the community - Secure inpatient and forensic mental health care for adults - The mental health of older adults - Section 3 - Physical health issues in mental health practice – CBTN - Psychodynamic and psychoanalytic therapeutic interventions in mental health - Recovery - Social inclusion - Conclusion

2009 368pp
ISBN-13: 978–0–335–23358–8   (ISBN-10: 033–5–23358–9) Paperback
ISBN-13: 978–0–335–23357–1   (ISBN-10: 033–5–23357–0) Hardback

PHYSICAL HEALTH AND WELL-BEING IN MENTAL HEALTH NURSING

Michael Nash

This groundbreaking book provides mental health nurses with the core knowledge of the physical health issues that they need for their work, and places these in a context that can be easily integrated into clinical practice. Michael Nash considers the risk factors and assessment priorities amongst different mental health client groups and provides clinical insights into how best to work with service users to ensure their health is assessed and improved.

Readers are encouraged to critically examine the notion that poor health in clients is solely related to lifestyle factors and how best they can contribute to better health outcomes for their clients.

The book includes coverage of:

- Core concepts of physical health/illness in mental illness
- Impacts of physical illness on people with severe mental illness
- Current practice issues and barriers to good physical health

Each chapter includes case studies, examples, diagrams and exercises for self-testing and reflection, which will help readers develop their own skills and practice.

Physical Health and Well-Being in Mental Health Nursing is a must-have text for students and practitioners working in mental health nursing. It is also useful reading for practice nurses, district nurses, midwives and all allied health practitioners.

Contents:

An introduction to physical health in mental illness - An introduction to key concepts in measuring health and illness - Clinical skills for physical assessment in mental health settings - Principles of physical health assessment in mental health care - Physical assessment: Assessing cardiovascular health - Assessing respiratory health in mental health - Assessing nutrition, diet and physical activity - Medication adverse drug reactions and physical health - Physical health emergencies in mental health settings - Practical steps in improving the physical health of people with severe mental illness

2009 232pp
ISBN-13: 978–0–335–23399–1 (ISBN-10: 033–5–23399–6) Paperback
ISBN-13: 978–0–335–23398–4 (ISBN-10: 033–5–23398–8) Hardback